GENITO-URINARY PROBLEMS

RN

NURSING ASSESSMENT SERIES

JOAN DOYLE, R.N., B.S.N.
NANCY REILLY, R.N., B.S.N., CURN

Series Editor
Margaret Van Meter, R.N.
Clinical Editor, RN Magazine

MEDICAL ECONOMICS BOOKS
Oradell, New Jersey 07649

Library of Congress Cataloging in Publication Data

Doyle, Joan.
    Genitourinary problems.

    (RN nursing assessment series; 6)
    Bibliography: p.
    Includes index.
    1. Urological nursing.   I. Reilly, Nancy, 1957-
II. Title.   III. Series: RN nursing assessment series;
v. 6.   [DNLM: 1. Genital Diseases, Male — nursing.
2. Urogenital System — nurses' instruction.   3. Urologic
Diseases — nursing.   WY   100   R627   1982   v.   6]
RC874.7.D69   1984   610.73'69   84-9144
ISBN 0-87489-286-4

Cover design by Jerry Wilke

ISBN 0-87489-286-4

Medical Economics Company Inc.
Oradell, New Jersey 07649

Printed in the United States of America

CONTENTS

PUBLISHER'S NOTES

Physical assessment is an integral part of the nursing process. Sharpening assessment skills, therefore, is bound to add logic and reason to planning, intervention, and evaluation. This volume in the *RN Nursing Assessment Series* focuses on assessment of genitourinary function. It provides norms against which to compare pathologic findings.

For easy access, an outline format combined with a clear, concise text — an organizational scheme that has proven popular with nurses — was adopted. The illustrations were selected specifically to add to the book's clarity and utility. Finally, the presentation of learning objectives and the inclusion of chapter quizzes, additional test questions, and a glossary make this book a learning/teaching tool.

Joan Doyle, R.N., B.S.N., is head nurse of the Urology Unit at the Hospital of the University of Pennsylvania. Nancy Reilly, R.N., B.S.N., C.U.R.N., is a urology nurse clinician at the same institution. In addition, she is coordinator of urology outpatient care, and participates in inservice education for staff nurses. Margaret Van Meter, R.N., the series editor, is *RN* Magazine's clinical editor for development and also serves as a private nurse consultant.

1

Anatomy and Physiology of the Genitourinary System

OBJECTIVES

After completing this chapter, you will be able to:

1. *Describe the basic anatomy of the urinary tract and male reproductive system*
2. *Explain urine production in terms of the structures involved*
3. *Trace the passage of urine from formation to excretion*
4. *Relate how ejaculatory products pass from formation to excretion.*

A. Kidney

1. Anatomic location

The kidneys (Figure 1-1) are two bean-shaped organs that lie on either side of the vertebral column, between the 12th thoracic and third lumbar vertebrae. They are retroperitoneal; that is, they are positioned behind and below the lining of the abdominal cavity. The left kidney is usually slightly higher than the right. In adults, kidneys are 10 to 12 cm long, 5 to 6 cm wide, and about 3 cm thick.

2. Structure

The distal border of each kidney is convex and the medial border concave (Figure 1-2). The concave side is called the hilus. This is where the ureter is attached, along with the major renal blood vessels, lymphatics, and nerves. Each kidney is enclosed in a fibrous capsule. The kidneys are held in place by perirenal fat and connective tissue called the renal fascia. The organ has three major areas: the cortex, the medulla, and the pelvis. Collectively, they are referred to as the renal parenchyma.

a. Cortex. The renal cortex lies underneath the fibrous capsule. Portions of the cortex extend into the medulla. These renal columns arch around and between medullary renal pyramids. Much of the kidney's arterial and venous blood circulates in these columns.

b. Medulla. The medulla contains eight to 18 renal pyramids. The bases of the pyramids face the periphery of the kidney, and the apices, or papillae, project toward the renal pelvis. Urine drains into the renal pelvis from numerous small openings in the papillae.

c. Pelvis. The main components of the renal pelvis are the major and minor calyces. These calyces are pouches that extend from the hilus to the papillae.

The papillae drain into the minor calyces, which lead into the major calyces. The renal pelvis narrows as it nears the hilus, becoming the proximal end of the ureter.

Figure 1-1   *Urinary tract (female);* reproduced from *Nursing Care of Patients With Urologic Diseases*, 4th edition; Winter CC and Morel A, CV Mosby Co., St. Louis, 1977.

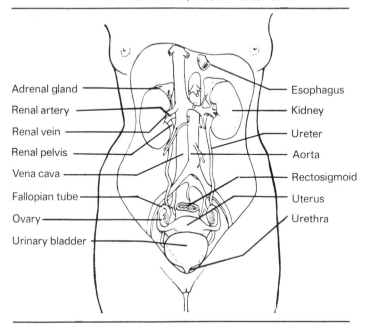

Adrenal gland — Esophagus
Renal artery — Kidney
Renal vein — Ureter
Renal pelvis — Aorta
Vena cava — Rectosigmoid
Fallopian tube — Uterus
Ovary — Urethra
Urinary bladder —

Figure 1-2   *Anatomy of the kidney*

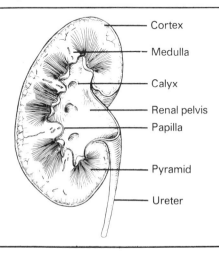

— Cortex
— Medulla
— Calyx
— Renal pelvis
— Papilla
— Pyramid
— Ureter

3. Nephron

The functional unit of the kidney is the nephron (Figure 1-3). Each kidney contains more than one million tubular nephrons, the site of urine production. The nephron uses filtration, reabsorption, and secretion to produce urine.

a. Structure. A nephron consists of a glomerulus, Bowman's capsule, and a tubule. Blood flows from afferent arterioles into the glomerulus, a clump of capillaries. High pressure in these vessels forces blood through a filtering membrane that separates blood contents from plasma. The filtrate flows into Bowman's capsule, which surrounds the glomerulus, and from there to the tubule, the site of reabsorption and secretion.

b. Function. Reabsorption pulls water, electrolytes, hormones, vitamins, and other useful substances out of the filtrate as it passes through the tubules. The remaining chemicals and waste products are secreted through the tubules. This modified filtrate has now become urine and passes from the tubules into the calyces, into the renal pelvis, then to the ureter.

Several factors, particularly the secretion of antidiuretic hormone (ADH) from the hypothalamus, affect the volume and concentration of urine. The secretion of ADH increases and decreases in response to the solute concentration of blood reaching the hypothalamus. Water loss by other systems, disease processes, alcohol consumption, and drugs – particularly diuretics – are other factors that affect the amount and concentration of urine.

4. Blood supply

The kidney receives its blood supply from the abdominal aorta via the large renal artery, which enters the kidney at the hilus. The renal artery branches into an intricate system of arteries – the interlobar arteries – which pass between the pyramids. The interlobar arteries run into the corticomedullary area, where they divide into the arcuate arteries at the bases of the renal pyramids. At the same place, the arcuate arteries branch into the interlobular arteries, some of which

Figure 1-3 *The nephron*

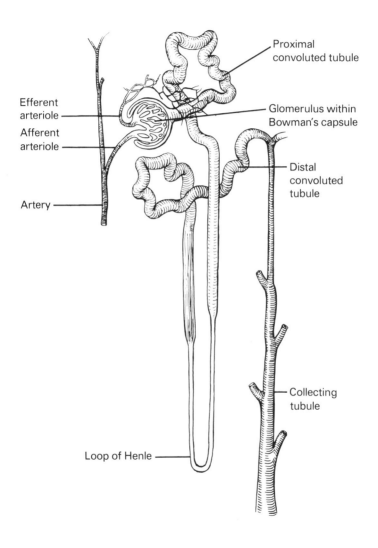

Proximal convoluted tubule

Efferent arteriole

Afferent arteriole

Glomerulus within Bowman's capsule

Distal convoluted tubule

Artery

Collecting tubule

Loop of Henle

supply the renal cortex and capsule while others give rise to the afferent arterioles, which become the glomeruli.

From the glomeruli, efferent arterioles carry blood into two important networks: the peritubular capillaries that surround the renal tubules and the vasa recta, a network of vessels that dip into the medulla and then return to the cortex. The peritubular network keeps the pressure high within the glomerulus. The function of the vasa recta is concentration.

5. Venous return

Venous blood leaves the kidney through a series of vessels corresponding to the arterial system; the interlobular veins drain into the arcuate veins at the bases of the pyramids. These, in turn, form the interlobar veins, which empty into the renal vein at the hilus. The renal vein then connects with the inferior vena cava.

6. Nerve supply

Both the parasympathetic and the sympathetic nervous systems innervate the kidney. Renal nerves enter the hilus along with the renal blood vessels. A denervated kidney can continue to form urine.

7. Other kidney functions

Production of urine is not the kidney's only function. Hormonal control of blood pressure, regulation of fluids and acid-base balance, degradation of insulin, synthesis of prostaglandins, red blood cell production, and metabolism of vitamin D are its other major functions.

B. Ureters

1. Structure and location

The ureters are two hollow tubes that carry urine from the kidneys to the bladder. In adults, ureters are 25 to 35 cm long. The proximal end of the ureter expands at the hilus to become the renal pelvis. It travels distally to enter the bladder on one or another side of its posterior aspect. The site of attachment of the ureter to the kidney is called the ureteropelvic junction. The ureterovesical junction is where the ureter joins the bladder.

The ureter has three layers: an inner mucosal layer lining the lumen, a middle muscular layer, and a fibrous outer layer. The muscular layer is mesh-like, with fibers running in many directions. The ureters are surrounded by abdominal muscles and the pelvic wall. They lie in connective tissue and fascia.

2. Function

Urine travels through the ureters by peristalsis. Peristaltic waves occur one to five times per minute. The muscular layer of the ureter performs these involuntary and regular contractions. The lumen of the ureter expands and contracts in response to peristalsis. The lumen is almost completely closed between intervals of urine passage, resembling a flat five-pointed star. As urine is pushed through the ureter, the lumen opens up to a full circle, as large as 2 mm in diameter.

3. Ureterovesical junction

How the ureter enters the bladder is particularly significant. Each ureter runs 1.5 to 2 cm past the bladder wall. This most distal portion of the ureter acts as a valve, preventing reflux of urine toward the kidney when the bladder contracts or is distended. This reflux can lead to serious urinary tract infections.

4. Blood supply

Arterial blood comes to the ureter from vessels that run along its length, with branching vessels feeding in and out of the ureter in several places. The renal and testicular or ovarian arteries contribute to the ureter's blood supply at the renal pelvis. Traveling distally, the aorta, the superior and inferior vesical arteries, the umbilical arteries, and the uterine arteries all provide ureteric branches. Each ureter has an increased blood supply as it nears the bladder. Venous drainage occurs in vessels paired with the ureteric arteries.

5. Nerve supply

Nerve supply to the ureter originates from the 11th thoracic to the first lumbar nerves.

C. Bladder

1. Location

The urinary bladder is a hollow muscular organ that lies in the anterior portion of the pelvis, behind the symphysis pubis and in front of the rectal septum. When empty, the bladder is flat. When distended, it ascends superiorly. Normally, it holds up to about 500 cc of urine, but, when maximally distended, the bladder can hold more than 1000 cc. In degenerative or neurogenic conditions, it may be limited to less than 100 cc. When the bladder is distended, it rises above the symphysis pubis and can be readily palpated. Severe distention causes the lower abdomen to bulge. Connective tissue between the symphysis pubis and the bladder allows for expansion.

2. Structures

The bladder is supported by a layer of loose fascia surrounding it and a ligament that extends from the bladder neck to the pelvic diaphragm. In males, this ligament is also attached to the base of the prostate. In males, the seminal vesicles and the vas deferens lie within the perivesical fascia. In females, the fundus of the bladder is attached loosely to the anterior wall of the vagina.

The innermost layer of the bladder wall is transitional epithelium. The middle portion is composed of three muscular layers. It is thought that the inner and outer muscular layers contain fibers that run longitudinally, while the middle muscular layer has circular fibers. This network of fibers makes up the detrusor muscle, which is responsible for the voluntary contraction of the bladder during voiding and for the elasticity that allows the bladder to expand. Muscle fibers thicken and become denser as they near the bladder neck, forming the theoretical internal sphincter that keeps the bladder neck closed until voiding.

Presuming a viewpoint inside the bladder, a triangle whose corners are the ureterovesical junctions and the internal sphincter can be imagined. This triangular area is known as the trigone. When visualized, it shows the firm attachment of the ureters to the bladder.

3. Bladder filling

The muscular bladder responds to increasing volume by adaptive stretching and intravesical pressure. This pressure remains relatively low and constant as urine accumulates. When distention occurs, intravesical pressure rises and stretch receptors in the bladder wall are stimulated, causing the desire to urinate, or urgency. If suppression of urgency is desired, external sphincter muscles in the pelvic floor are voluntarily contracted. When the volume of urine is not great, intravesical pressure will decrease. At larger volumes, urgency can't be suppressed with pressure inside the bladder continuing to rise. Numerous factors affect an individual's adaptation to bladder volume and urgency, including habit, stress, and certain drugs.

4. Bladder emptying

Sensation of urgency is an involuntary manifestation of the bladder's nerve supply and stretch receptors. Initiation of voiding – also called urination or micturition – is normally voluntary, the result of a highly complex neurologic phenomenon involving sympathetic and parasympathetic nerve signals from the spinal cord and the brain to the bladder. These neurologic impulses cause the bladder to contract while the internal and external sphincters simultaneously open or relax.

Pressure inside the bladder rises sharply as it contracts, propelling urine through the bladder neck and urethra. Valves at the junction of the ureters and the bladder prevent urine from flowing back into the ureters (reflux) despite the increase in intravesical pressure.

After voiding, the now-flattened bladder resumes a low intravesical pressure while urethral sphincters contract once again to maintain continence while the bladder fills again with urine.

5. Nerve supply

Nerve supply to the bladder is an intricate and complex system. The primary center for voiding is located in the sacral spinal cord; the cerebral cortex is also known to play a role in the initiation of voiding.

Innervation of the bladder involves the hypogastric, pelvic, and pudendal nerves. The parasympathetic and sympathetic nervous systems ensure that the bladder, urethra, and urethral sphincters act in coordination in retaining and voiding urine.

6. Blood supply

Arterial blood to the bladder comes mainly through the superior and inferior vesical arteries. The superior vesical artery arises from the umbilical and internal iliac arteries and supplies the superior portion of the bladder. The inferior vesical artery, which may be a branch of the middle rectal artery, supplies the inferior portion of the bladder. A network of veins surrounding the bladder eventually enters into the hypogastric veins.

D. Urethra

The urethra resembles a tube-like structure that originates at the base of the bladder and extends to an opening at the body surface.

1. Female urethra

In the adult female, the urethra is 3 to 4 cm long and 8 mm in diameter. It is slightly curved, with its external orifice (meatus) located between the labia minora and anterior to the vagina. No portion of the female urethra is external to the body trunk.

The lining of the female urethra is transitional epithelium, which contains mucus-secreting glands; the submucosa consists of connective and elastic tissue. The external sphincter is formed from a circular muscle layer, which is continuous with the bladder.

Urethral blood supply is from the inferior vesical and vaginal arteries.

2. Male urethra

The male urethra is a long, curved, narrow tube about 20 cm long and 8 to 9 mm in diameter (Figure 1-4). It is used for the passage of urine and ejaculatory products to the outside. The male urethra can be divided into three main parts: the prostatic urethra, the membranous urethra, and the cavernous urethra.

Figure 1-4 *Male bladder and urethra;* from Lerner J, Kahn Z: *Mosby's Manual of Urologic Nursing.* St. Louis: Mosby, 1982.

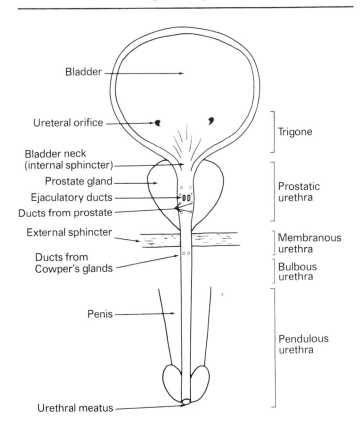

a. Prostatic urethra. This part of the urethra is approximately 3 cm in length and extends below the bladder neck through the prostate gland to the pelvic floor. The ejaculatory ducts, which carry spermatic fluid, open into the posterior wall of the prostatic urethra.

b. Membranous urethra. This section is 1 to 2 cm in length and ends at the external sphincter.

c. Cavernous urethra. Also known as the penile urethra, the cavernous urethra is approximately 16 cm long and is the distal portion of the urethra. It extends through the penis to the urethral orifice located at the tip of the penis.

Urethral mucosa is composed of epithelium, with its submucosa containing connective and elastic tissue and smooth muscle. Several glands (Cowper's glands) open into the male urethra where they secrete an alkaline fluid that aids in the motility and preservation of the sperm.

E. Prostate gland

1. Structure

The prostate is a fibromuscular and glandular organ that lies inferior to the bladder (see Figure 1-4). Its apex rests on the urogenital diaphragm and the sphincter urethrae muscle, and its base at the neck of the bladder. In the adult male, the normal prostate measures 4 to 6 cm and weighs 15 to 20 grams. Its contact with the rectal wall allows the gland to be palpated. The prostate is divided into five lobes: the anterior, posterior, middle, right lateral, and left lateral.

The urethra enters the prostate near the middle of the base of the gland and leaves the anterior surface above the apex. The ejaculatory ducts enter at the posterior border of the base and pass obliquely downward and forward and converge in the urethra.

2. Function

The prostate contains many glands throughout its musculature. These glands manufacture a secretion that becomes part of the ejaculate. This secretion supplies nutrients to the sperm and aids in their passage.

3. Blood and nerve supply

The blood supply to the prostate comes from the inferior vesical, internal pudendal, and middle hemorrhoidal arteries. The prostate is innervated by the pudendal nerves.

F. Scrotum

1. Structure

The scrotum is a pouch-like structure divided in halves by a septum of connective tissue. Each half contains a testis with its epididymis and spermatic cord (Figure 1-5).

The two layers of the scrotum are the skin and the tunica dartos. The skin of the scrotum, which is extremely thin and deeply pigmented, is separated by a median raphe that extends from the undersurface of the penis along the entire scrotum to the anus. The tunica dartos is the underlying connective tissue and separates the halves of the scrotum internally.

2. Function

In addition to supporting the testes, the scrotum aids in regulating their temperature by relaxing and contracting its muscle layer.

3. Arterial blood and nerve supply

Blood supply to the scrotum comes from the femoral, internal pudendal and inferior epigastric arteries. Innervation to the skin of the scrotum is by the ileoinguinal and external spermatic nerves. The pudendal branch of the posterior femoral and cutaneous and superficial perineal branches of the internal pudendal nerves supply the scrotum from the perineum.

G. Testes

The testes are paired oval structures suspended in the scrotum by the spermatic cord (see Figure 1-5). The average testicle is 4 to 5 cm in length, 3 cm wide, and about 2 cm thick. It is within the testes that sperm (spermatozoa) are formed.

Figure 1-5 *Male genitourinary tract*

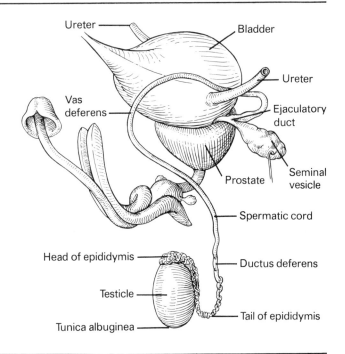

1. Structure

The epididymis is attached to the posterior border of the testis where it caps the testis with its head. The testis is covered by a thick external covering, the tunica albuginea, made up of dense, white fibrous connective tissue. The tunica albuginea radiates into the interior of the testis, forming 600-1200 seminiferous tubules with a combined length of one mile. The seminiferous tubules enter the mediastinum testis and anastamose in a network of epithelial lined channels in the fibrous stroma that make up the rete testis. The seminiferous tubules are coiled (ductuli contorti) in the cortex of the testis and unite with each other to form straight connecting canals (ductuli recti), which open into the efferent ducts that drain the formed sperm into the epididymis.

2. Epididymis

The epididymis is a sausage- or comma-shaped structure, about 2 inches in length, attached to the posterior lateral surface of the testis. The epididymis is divided into three parts: the head (globus major), which rests on the upper pole of the testis; the body (corpus); and the tail (globus minor). The head of the epididymis is connected to the testis by efferent ducts from the testis. The body of the epididymis, which is attached to the posterior surface of the testis, contains a mass of coiled ducts, as does the head. The ducts of the epididymis become thicker and wider in the tail portion to become continuous with the vas deferens that join other vessels to form the spermatic cord.

Sperm formed in the testes pass into the epididymis, through the vas deferens to the seminal vesicles, and then into the prostatic urethra via the ejaculatory ducts.

3. Blood supply

Arterial blood supply to the testes and epididymis is from the internal spermatic arteries, which then join with the vasa arteries that branch off the hypogastric artery. The epididymis has an additional blood supply from the vasa arteries.

H. Penis

1. Structure

The penis is a cylindrical erectile organ predominately used for sexual function. It contains a pathway for urine passage. The penis consists of three elongated cavernous masses, two corpora cavernosa and the corpus spongiosum (which contains the urethra), richly supplied with blood vessels and having sympathetic innervation. Each corpus is enclosed in a fascious sheath (tunica albuginea) and together they are surrounded by a thick fibrous envelope called Buck's fascia.

The corpora cavernosa lie next to each other on the dorsum of the penis, parallel to the urethra, while the spongiosum rests in the ventral groove and surrounds the urethra. The distal portion of the corpus spongiosum is expanded to form the glans penis, a cone-shaped structure on which the urethral meatus opens.

The skin of the penis is dark, hairless, thin, and loose, allowing for distention. The prepuce of foreskin covers the glans at the base.

2. Function

Erection is caused by engorgement of the cavernous chambers with blood. Sensory impulses lead to vasodilation of the arteries of the corpora, opening of the arteriovenous shunts, and inhibition of venous outflow.

3. Blood supply

Arterial blood supply to the penis is from the internal pudendal arteries, which branch off to supply the cavernous and spongy bodies, the glans penis, and the urethra.

I. Spermatic cord

The spermatic cord is a fascia-covered structure that consists of the ductus deferens, the deferential artery and vein, the testicular artery, lymphatics, and nerves. The spermatic cord suspends the testicle in the scrotum. Contained within the spermatic cord is the ductus deferens, a thick-walled tube that begins in the epididymis and extends to the prostate, where it joins with the duct of the seminal vesicle and becomes the ejaculatory duct. Surrounding the vessels of the cord and the vas deferens is the cremaster muscle, which is responsible for the length of the spermatic cord and determines the distance of the testes from the body.

Blood supply to the spermatic cord is derived from the deferential artery and the external spermatic artery.

J. Seminal vesicles and ejaculatory ducts

The seminal vesicles are paired lobulated pouches that secrete an alkaline fluid believed essential to the preservation and transportation of the sperm. Somewhere near the prostatic base, the duct from the seminal vesicles joins the duct from the vas deferens to become the ejaculatory duct. The ejaculatory ducts empty into the prostatic urethra.

Blood is supplied to these structures from the deferential artery as a branch of the inferior vesical artery. Innervation to the seminal vesicles come mainly from the sympathetic nerve plexus.

QUIZ

1. The ureter is attached to the kidney at the area known as the _____.

2. Urine is formed in the _____, the tubular structures found within the kidney.

3. The major artery providing renal circulation is the

   _____.

4. The nephron uses the following processes in the production of urine: _____, _____, and _____.

5. The muscle in the bladder that contracts during urination is the _____ muscle.

6. The male and female urethra have these histologic characteristics in common:

   _____

   _____

7. _____, _____, and _____ are the three main parts of the male urethra.

8. The _____ ducts enter the prostate at its base and converge in the urethra.

9. The _____, _____, and _____ are structures within the scrotum.

10. The site of sperm formation is the _____.

ANSWERS

1. Hilus.

2. Nephron.

3. Renal artery.

4. Reabsorption, filtration, secretion.

5. Detrusor.

6. Both are composed of transitional epithelium.
Both have a circular muscle layer continuous with the bladder.

7. Prostatic, membranous, cavernous.

8. Ejaculatory.

9. Testes, epididymis, spermatic cord.

10. Testis.

C H A P T E R

The Genitourinary History

OBJECTIVES

After completing this chapter, you will be able to:

1. Ask the patient questions appropriate to the genitourinary tract history

2. Describe the effects of other body systems on the genitourinary tract

3. List the psychological factors that can influence your ability to obtain a thorough history

4. Describe the symptoms that commonly affect the genitourinary tract.

A. Rationale for the genitourinary nursing history

Assessment of the genitourinary tract is an important part of the overall physical assessment of the patient. And no physical assessment is complete without an accurate nursing history. This is true of all patients receiving nursing care, not just of patients whose primary problem is a disorder of the genitourinary tract. For this latter group, however, particular emphasis should be placed on obtaining information relevant to the problem. Information on the patient's previous medical history is also important, as many diseases or injuries of other body systems may ultimately affect the genitourinary tract.

For a patient whose primary disorder is not of the genitourinary tract, information regarding voiding, renal function, and the reproductive organs has value in assessing potential problems that may arise during or interfere with the patient's evaluation and treatment.

B. The genitourinary nursing history

1. General health history

Ask the patient questions about his or her overall medical history, including currently treated health problems, previous hospitalizations for treatment or surgical procedures (including dates), and health problems for which the patient has sought medical care in the past. Find out whether these problems are now resolved and, if so, how and when did they get resolved.

a. Present functioning. Question the patient regarding present functioning of body systems; determine if the patient has any complaint specific to one system or related to several systems. If a problem is undiagnosed or if the patient has not previously sought medical advice for it, find out what is the patient's opinion as to its cause.

b. Medications. Determine what, if any, medications the patient takes, both regularly and prn (include dosages and frequency). This is of particular importance in the patient with voiding dysfunction.

c. Allergies. Find out whether the patient has any allergy. An allergy to iodine or shellfish or any previous hypersensitivity to X-ray contrast material is important, as many genitourinary diagnostic tests involve the use of such material.

2. Genitourinary history

Tables 2-1 to 2-4 summarize specific information that should be included in a detailed genitourinary history. They will help you to ask pertinent questions. The patient, family members, or significant others may be the source of your information.

TABLE 2-1

RENAL HISTORY

Hypertension: How long? Any medications to control it?

Bleeding tendencies?

Pruritus?

Fever, chills, night sweats?

Numbness or tingling of extremities?

Fluid losses: Increased urine production (polyuria), heavy perspiration, weight loss? Decreased urine production (oliguria)?

Gastrointestinal symptoms: Nausea, vomiting, diarrhea, anorexia?

Congenital kidney disorders: How treated or corrected?

Pyelonephritis: History of kidney infection? How often? How treated?

History of stone disease: Any stones passed? When? Any previous surgery for stone disease? Any dietary restrictions?

Recent blunt trauma to flank area: Athletic injury, accident, fall, struck with blunt object?

Hematuria: Microscopic or gross (bright red urine)? Any clots?

Pain: Where? One or both sides? Constant or intermittent? Sharp and stabbing or dull and aching: What brings it on or relieves it? Does it radiate? Where?

TABLE 2-2

URETERAL HISTORY

Congenital ureteral disorders: How treated or corrected?

History of stone disease: Any previous ureteral stones removed surgically?

Blunt trauma: Recent injury to ureteral area? Recent surgery?

Pain: Back pain or abdominal pain? In females: Genital, labial pain? In males: Genital, testicular pain?

TABLE 2-3

VOIDING HISTORY

Suprapubic pain: Constant or occasional? Associated with voiding only or with bladder filling?

History of recurrent cystitis: How treated? How often?

Dysuria: Burning on urination?

Nocturia: Awakening at night to void?

Frequency: Frequent voiding during the day? How often?

Urgency: Sudden, strong desire to void?

Intermittency: Voiding in spurts or intermittent stream?

Decreased force of stream: Does it take longer than usual to empty the bladder?

Hesitancy: Does it take a long time to begin voiding despite a desire to void?

Terminal dribbling: Does urine dribble for a minute or longer after voiding?

Retention, inability to void: Sudden and painful? Situational?

Incontinence:

    Enuresis: Bedwetting? With or without awakening?

    Stress: Leakage of urine during coughing, laughing, jumping, straining?

    Urge: Unable to get to toilet or urinal before voiding begins?

    Total: Constant, continuous loss of urine?

Hematuria: Microscopic or gross?

Previous prostate surgery: Abdominal or transurethral? When?

Previous female reproductive history: Number of children delivered vaginally? Recurrent vaginal infections? Method of birth control?

TABLE 2-4

MALE GENITOSEXUAL HISTORY

Scrotal swelling: How severe? How long?

Testicular mass: When discovered?

Testicular pain?

Prostate pain: Deep pain intensified by sitting?

Hematospermia: Blood in semen?

Retrograde ejaculation (semen discharges into bladder instead of out urethra): Cloudy urine?

Infertility?

Impotence?

a. Symptomatology. When gathering information about the patient's symptoms, be sure to include when the symptoms began, any precipitating factors, and any progression or worsening of the symptoms since they began.

In some cases, the patient may be relatively asymptomatic. The problem may have been discovered incidentally, during a general medical examination or during evaluation of a different problem. Ask the patient how he or she discovered the problem and how long ago.

b. Diagnostic studies. After completing your history, you may want to begin preparing the patient for diagnostic studies. It is never too early to teach and reassure the patient about studies involving the genitourinary tract. Providing the patient with honest and consistent information may help to allay fears and embarrassment.

3. Psychological factors

Keep in mind that voiding is a very personal thing. It may be embarrassing and uncomfortable for the patient to be questioned about problems with his or her urinary tract. Make every attempt to make the patient comfortable with you; provide for privacy during questioning and be discreet about the manner in which you interview the patient.

a. Sensitivity about sex. Questions regarding sexual function may be especially humiliating for the patient and difficult for you to ask. Approaching this subject with a professional but caring attitude will help you to obtain the necessary information. Be aware of nonverbal clues that may help you to ascertain the patient's reaction to questioning and his or her honesty in answering.

b. Anxiety. Try to determine if the patient is anxious or nervous. People who are excessively anxious may have difficulty voiding in public situations, as may people who experienced psychological trauma during toilet training.

As with other body systems, the genitourinary tract may be the target area of a stress response, resulting in pain or difficulties voiding. Recognition of the patient's normal state of anxiety will help you to develop an effective plan of care.

QUIZ

1. Diseases or disorders of _____ may ultimately affect the genitourinary tract.

2. Allergy to _____ or _____ is of particular importance in the patient with a genitourinary problem.

3. It is important to determine the _____ and _____ of the patient's problem.

4. Providing the patient with _____ and _____ information helps to ease fears about diagnostic studies.

5. _____ during questioning will help to make the patient feel _____ about answering.

6. _____ patients may be particularly prone to have voiding difficulties.

7. Testicular pain may be pain referred from the _____.

8. Pain on urination is called _____.

9. Nocturia means _____ _____.

10. Inability to void is called _____.

ANSWERS

1. Other body systems.
2. Iodine, shellfish.
3. Origin, symptoms.
4. Honest, consistent.
5. Privacy, comfortable.
6. Anxious.
7. Ureter.
8. Dysuria.
9. Awakening from sleep to void.
10. Retention.

C H A P T E R

General Physical Assessment

OBJECTIVES

After completing this chapter, you will be able to:

1. *Perform inspection, palpation, percussion, and auscultation of the kidney*
2. *Examine the penis, scrotum, and testes and list normal and any abnormal findings*
3. *Describe the pelvic examination*
4. *Teach patients what is involved in the physical examination of the genitourinary system whether it is performed by a physician or a nurse.*

Figure 3-1 *Palpation of bladder*

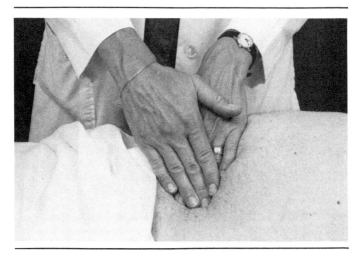

In most settings, the physician is primarily responsible for the physical examination. The nurse's role is to assist the physician and support the patient. Since most genitourinary examinations are embarrassing to the patient and may cause anxiety, you should explain the procedures prior to the exam and answer any question the patient may have concerning it.

A. Examination of male and female patients

1. Kidney

a. Inspection. Inspection should include examination of the skin on the abdomen and flank for abnormal findings such as ulcerations or discolorations. Observe this area also for any mass. The normal kidney is usually not detectable on inspection, but a tumor, abscess, or cyst may cause bulging in the flank.

b. Palpation. Because of the kidney's location in the abdominal cavity, palpation is difficult, especially in obese or muscular patients. Have the patient lie supine on a firm surface. With one hand on the costovertebral angle (where

Figure 3-2 *Percussion of bladder*

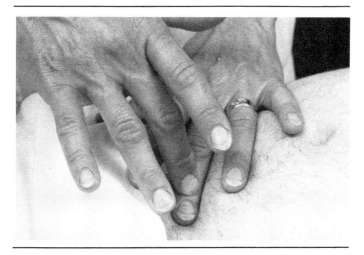

the ribs articulate with the vertebrae) and the other hand on the patient's abdomen, just below the costal margin, palpate the lower pole of the kidney on deep inspiration by the patient. On inspiration, the kidney moves downward and is easier to trap at that point. The kidney may also be palpated by the "capture" technique. With your hands in the same position on the patient, instruct the patient to inhale deeply. On inspiration, press your hands together. As the patient exhales, you will feel the kidney between your hands.

c. Percussion. With the patient in a sitting position, place your palm over the costovertebral angle and then gently strike that hand with your other in a fist. Assess the patient for any tenderness or pain over the area of the blow.

d. Auscultation. A systolic bruit may be heard over the costovertebral area and upper quadrants, although this is abnormal. Renal artery stenosis or an aneurysm may cause a bruit.

2. Bladder

A normal bladder can be palpated (Figure 3-1) and percussed (Figure 3-2) only when it contains 150 ml or more of urine.

More than 500 ml of urine in the bladder will cause the bladder to bulge or appear distended in the suprapubic area of a lean patient. Percussion will help detect a distended bladder in a patient with a large abdomen. A distended bladder sounds dull to percussion, and an empty bladder sounds tympanic.

B. Examination of male patients

1. Penis

The penis is best inspected with the examiner seated and the patient standing. Inspect the penis for size, color, shape, and any lesion or inflammation. At the same time, inspect the groin for lumps or skin discoloration. If the patient is not circumcised, retract the foreskin and inspect for swelling, discharge, or cracking of the skin, which would be indicative of an infection. Retraction of the foreskin may also reveal tumors. Examine the shape and size of the urethral meatus. Any discharge or swelling in this area is a significant finding. Send for culture a specimen of any discharge from the penis.

Palpate the penis from the perineum to the tip for plaques (which are present in Peyronie's disease) or masses.

2. Scrotum and testes

After examining the penis, proceed, with the patient in the same position, to examine the scrotum and testes.

a. Inspection. Inspect the scrotum for any lesion or inflammation. The scrotal skin is frequently the site for sebaceous cysts, which may be found on inspection.

b. Palpation. Palpate the testes between the fingers and thumb. They should feel firm and move freely in the scrotal sac. Any hardened area in a testis may indicate a malignancy and should be explored further. Any difference in weight should be noted, as a testicle with a malignancy usually weighs more than the other.

Palpate the epididymis for any swelling or tenderness. The normal epididymis usually adheres closely to the testes and its entire length can be palpated.

c. Transillumination. Transillumination may be performed on any scrotal masses to determine if the mass is solid, as with a tumor, or if it is transilluminable, which would indicate a cyst or hydrocele.

3. Prostate

Palpation of the prostate is done during the rectal examination. The rectal exam may be performed with the patient either standing and bending over the examining table or lying on his side with his back to you and knees up toward his chin.

a. Findings. Insert a well lubricated gloved finger into the rectum. Note sphincter tone and feel for hemorrhoids or lesions. The normal prostate is about the size of a walnut and should feel firm and symmetrical. Any hard or indurated areas should be further evaluated, as these usually indicate a cancerous growth. Any bogginess or enlargement of the gland can indicate benign prostatic hypertrophy.

b. Prostatic massage. Prostatic massage will cause some prostatic secretions to be expressed out the urethral meatus. These should be sent for examination. Never carry out a prostatic massage on patients with acute prostatitis or known prostatic cancer.

C. Examination of female patients

Most females with genitourinary problems require a thorough pelvic examination to rule out any contributing gynecological disorders. The pelvic exam and inspection of the external genitalia are best done with the patient on an examining table with her feet up in stirrups. Inspect the external genitalia for any abnormality. Note the skin color of the labia and examine the area for redness, swelling, uneven pigmentation, or lesions. Any discharge from the urethra or vagina should be sent for culture. A manual examination of the vaginal walls is done to detect irregularities and rule out cystocele. A speculum is then passed into the vagina to complete the vaginal exam and examine the cervix. A Pap smear may be obtained at this time.

QUIZ

1. Renal palpation is best performed with the patient _____ on a firm surface, while renal percussion is carried out with the patient in a _____ position.

2. A normal bladder can be palpated and percussed only when it contains _____ ml of urine. More than _____ ml of urine in the bladder will cause the bladder to bulge in the suprapubic area.

3. The penis should be inspected for _____, _____, _____, _____, and _____.

4. The testis should feel _____, and _____ _____ in the scrotal sac.

5. A testicle with a malignancy will weigh _____ than the other testicle.

6. _____ may be performed on any scrotal masses to determine if the mass is solid or transilluminable.

7. The prostate is examined by _____ exam and should feel _____ and _____.

8. Females with genitourinary problems usually require a thorough _____ exam.

9. Inspection of the female external genitalia is best done with the patient on the _____ with feet up in stirrups.

ANSWERS

1. Supine, sitting.

2. 150, 500.

3. Size, color, shape, lesions, inflammations.

4. Firm, move freely.

5. More.

6. Transillumination.

7. Rectal, firm, symmetrical.

8. Pelvic.

9. Exam table.

CHAPTER

4

Congenital Disorders of the Genitourinary Tract

OBJECTIVES

After completing this chapter, you will be able to:

1. *Describe the most common congenital anomalies of the genitourinary tract*

2. *Recognize the signs and symptoms of genitourinary tract congenital anomalies in the neonate*

3. *Describe the surgical procedures necessary to correct these anomalies*

4. *Care for the neonate with a genitourinary congenital anomaly with an understanding of the anatomic structures involved*

5. *Outline the special needs of parents of children with genitourinary anomalies*

Ten to 15 percent of all people are born with at least one genitourinary congenital anomaly. Many of these anomalies are so slight that they are virtually undetectable on physical examination of the neonate and may never present any difficulty throughout a normal life. Some anomalies create problems as the child grows into adulthood. Severe disorders are obvious at birth and require immediate surgical intervention.

Although knowledge of the embryologic development of the genitourinary tract is helpful in understanding the origins of these anomalies, embryology is not covered in this chapter. You can go to the selected readings for sources of information on embryology. This chapter describes the congenital anomalies that most frequently occur in the genitourinary tract, their anatomic consequences, symptoms, and methods of treatment or correction.

Remember that nursing care of the infant with a congenital defect includes the parents and family. This is a very stressful time for family members. Often they experience a kind of grieving as they mourn the birth of an abnormal child. Consistent communication between members of the health-care team and the infant's family helps to ease fears about diagnostic studies, surgery, and the potential for a normal life for the child.

A. Disorders of the kidney

1. Anomalies of number

a. Renal agenesis. Bilateral renal agenesis is the most severe of all urinary tract anomalies and is incompatible with life. The neonate's chest is compressed, and oligohydramnios is present, the result of no urine formation. Unilateral agenesis is far more common than bilateral and can be compatible with life, depending on the condition of the solitary kidney. There is, however, a great incidence of anomalies of the solitary kidney.

b. Extra kidney. This is extremely rare, resulting from a splitting of the embryologic origins of the kidney during fetal development. The third kidney has its own ureter, which may enter the bladder separately or join the ureter of the ipsilateral kidney. This anomaly is asymptomatic and usually not discovered unless other anomalies of the kidneys coexist. Diagnosis is made by intravenous pyelogram.

2. Anomalies of position

a. Ectopic kidney. This disorder results from a failure of a kidney to rise to its normal position in the retroperitoneal cavity. In most cases, the kidney can be found in the pelvis (Figure 4-1). Often ureteric anomalies are associated with ectopic kidney. The major difficulty with an ectopic kidney occurs in females during labor, when the kidney's position in the pelvis causes pain.

Figure 4-1 *Ectopic kidney located in pelvis;* Figures 4-1 through 4-6 from Lapides J: *Fundamentals of Urology.* Philadelphia: Saunders, 1979.

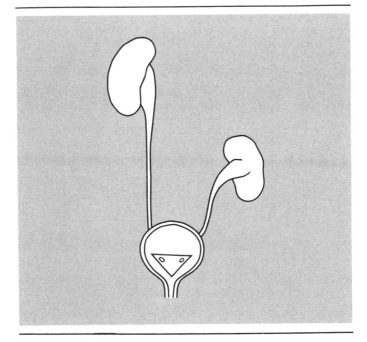

Figure 4-2 *Crossed renal ectopia*

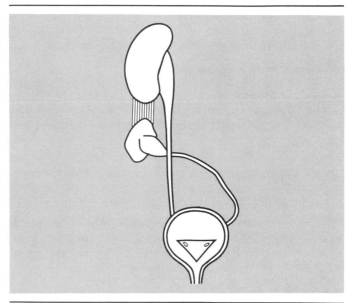

Figure 4-3 *Horseshoe kidney*

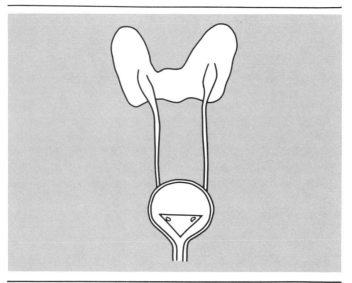

b. Crossed renal ectopia. In this condition, both kidneys are on the same side of the abdomen (Figure 4-2). It occurs when one kidney crosses the midline during fetal development. In many cases, the ectopic kidney fuses with the normal kidney. The ureters enter the bladder in the normal position. Clinically, this condition is asymptomatic.

3. Anomalies of development

a. Renal hypoplasia. This failure of the kidney to reach normal size is probably caused by a defect in the fetal development of the kidney's blood supply. This condition is common and can be asymptomatic. In some individuals, hypoplasia of the kidney has been linked to hypertension, in which case nephrectomy may be considered if conservative management of the hypertension fails. Whenever nephrectomy is a possibility, the remaining kidney's function must be carefully evaluated.

b. Horseshoe kidney. In horseshoe kidney, the lower poles of the two kidneys fuse during fetal development, forming one large kidney with two pelvises and two ureters (Figure 4-3). The kidney lies in the lower lumbar region. This renal anomaly may also be asymptomatic; however, its incidence is usually accompanied by other congenital disorders. When horseshoe kidney is the only anomaly, there is an increased chance of renal calculi and infection.

4. Cystic anomalies

a. Infantile polycystic kidneys. This is a very rare congenital birth defect. It is always bilateral, commonly causing death during the early days or months of life. The interstitial portion of the kidney's collecting tubules undergoes hyperplasia during development. The infant has abdominal masses, uremia, and signs of portal hypertension. Renal transplantation is the only treatment. This disease is an autosomal recessive trait.

b. Multicystic kidney. The multicystic kidney is nonfunctional and presents as an abdominal mass. It can occur unilaterally or bilaterally. If bilateral, the disease is incompatible with life. If unilateral and if the unaffected kidney is normal, the prognosis is excellent. This disease is not hereditary.

c. Adult polycystic kidney. Adult polycystic kidney disease results from the displacement of nephrons by cysts in the glomerular and tubular areas of the kidney. In most cases, this disease is unilateral, although it may occur bilaterally. The development and growth of these cysts compromises renal function. Symptoms do not appear until adulthood, when the disease usually begins, although children may be affected. Abdominal masses may be present. Diagnosis is made by intravenous pyelogram. Transplantation is necessary if renal function is poor. Genetically, this disease is an autosomal dominant trait. In some patients, it may also affect the liver.

5. Vascular anomalies

Additional renal arteries are common, as are extra renal veins, which occur more commonly on the left side. These present no problem unless venous abnormalities underlie failure of the kidney to ascend during development or obstruct the ureteropelvic junction. Aneurysms and arteriovenous malformations may also occur. Diagnosis is made by renal arteriography. Large renal arteriovenous malformations can lead to congestive heart failure, requiring surgical correction.

B. Disorders of the renal pelvis

1. Ureteropelvic junction obstruction

During fetal development, the renal pelvis forms at the distal end of the ureter. Several defective processes — including fibrous, vascular, or intrinsic — can lead to obstruction of the pelvis. The result is hydronephrosis, which appears physically in the infant as an abdominal mass. In children, pain and recurrent urinary tract infection are common. Diagnosis is made by intravenous pyelogram. Treatment is by surgical removal of the obstruction and reanastomosis of the ureter and renal pelvis, called pyeloplasty.

2. Duplication of the pelvis and ureter

This is a very common anomaly, which can range from the development of two separate pelvises and ureters in one kidney to a bifid pelvis, one that is split into two parts. The position of the ureters varies. Two separate ureters may drain the upper and lower portions of the kidney and enter the bladder separately, or the ureters may join together at some point between the kidney and bladder.

Symptoms vary, depending on the location and extent of the anomaly. If the anomaly creates an obstruction, resort to surgical intervention, such as reimplantation of the ureter into the bladder (ureteroneocystostomy), heminephrectomy, or removal of one ureter (ureterectomy), may be required.

C. Disorders of the ureter

1. Ectopic ureter

Occurring more frequently in females than in males, ectopic ureter results in problems similar to those described under duplication of the pelvis and ureter. In females, an extra ureter may develop and empty into the vagina or lower urethra, causing dribbling incontinence. Lower-pole ectopic ureters tend to result in vesicoureteric reflux. The results of such reflux may be infection and hydronephrosis. If two separate ureters exist, instead of fusing, they may cross before entering the bladder.

Treatment depends on the location of the ectopic ureter. Vaginal or urethral ureteral orifices can be surgically corrected by ureteroneocystostomy. This surgery may also be necessary for a ureter that refluxes. If there are no symptoms, no treatment is necessary.

2. Retrocaval ureter

In this anomaly, one ureter crosses the inferior vena cava before entering the bladder, assuming an S-shaped curve in order to do so (Figure 4-4). The result can be partial obstruction of the mid-ureter, which may require surgical division of the ureter with reanastomosis.

Figure 4-4 *Retrocaval ureter*

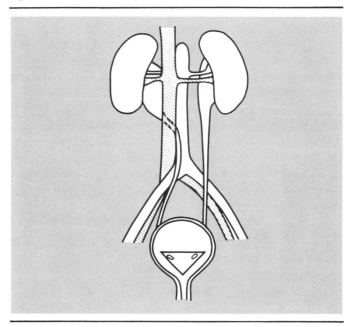

D. Disorders of the bladder

1. Exstrophy of the bladder

Exstrophy of the bladder is a serious congenital defect with several other anomalies of the genitourinary tract as well as other body systems. During fetal development, the mesoderm, which normally matures to cover the lower abdominal wall, fails to do so, the rectus muscles of the abdomen do not meet, and the pubic bones separate.

a. Appearance. In the infant born with classic exstrophy, the posterior wall of the bladder is everted outside the abdominal wall. Since the ureteric orifices enter the bladder at the posterior wall, these, too, are outside the body. Frequently, epispadias of the urethra is also present, as are bilateral hernias and often cryptorchidism in males. The penis is short and stubby in the more severe cases.

The severity of this anomaly can range from a mild musculoskeletal defect, which is almost undetectable and is easily corrected, to the classic total exstrophy-epispadias complex with numerous anomalies.

In females with exstrophy, the labia are separated, and the clitoris is bifid. The urethra is epispadiac and may be difficult to find. Abnormalities of the size and position of the vagina may be present, and anomalies of the uterus and cervix may also occur.

b. Associated disorders. The infant born with classic exstrophy is totally incontinent. The upper urinary tract is most often normal. Hydronephrosis and hydroureters occur only when the exstrophy is so mild that it goes untreated. In these children, the defect is discovered only when symptoms of renal obstruction occur.

Anomalies of other systems frequently seen along with bladder exstrophy are club feet, cleft palate, rectovaginal fistula, and imperforate anus.

c. Treatment. Treatment of bladder exstrophy varies with the severity of the anomaly. Those with very mild exstrophy, sometimes referred to as pseudoexstrophy, have only a mild musculoskeletal defect that requires no treatment. The urinary tract functions normally. The widened pelvic bones cause a waddling gait in young children, which is self-correcting as they grow. In classic exstrophy-epispadias, surgical intervention is necessary. Closure of the abdominal wall and reconstruction of the urethra is possible in some cases, resulting in normal function. In others, supravesical urinary diversion is performed. Ureterosigmoidostomy was at one time the preferred form of diversion. In this procedure, the ureters are surgically implanted into the sigmoid colon, and a rectal pouch is created. The child then learns to void out the rectum. Electrolyte imbalances are common after ureterosigmoidostomy, and it is now rarely performed. Cutaneous ureterostomy, in which the ureters are brought out to the abdominal wall, or ureteroileostomy (ileal conduit) are other common methods of urinary diversion. Correction of epispadias is explained on page 43.

As with all children born with congenital defects, nurses play an important role in comforting the parents and caring for the child who undergoes surgery. These parents need special understanding and teaching so they can care for their infant at home.

2. Patent urachus

The urachus is a cord that extends from the apex of the bladder to the umbilicus during fetal development. Normally, it closes and becomes a supporting ligament for the bladder. In patent urachus, this fails to occur. It is easily detectable, as urine discharges from the umbilicus during voiding. Often, the urethra is obstructed. To correct this anomaly, the urethral obstruction is corrected, and the urachus closed.

E. Disorders of the urethra and penis

1. Epispadias

This is an extremely rare anomaly, occurring even more rarely in females than in males. Because the embryologic development of the urethra is of the same origin as the bladder, epispadias is usually seen along with bladder exstrophy. It can, however, be present by itself.

a. In males. Epispadias in males results from failure of the urethra to close during fetal development. Instead, the urinary opening extends along some length of the dorsal side of the penis. It is classified into three types, depending on the extent of the opening:

- balanic or glandular epispadias, in which the opening extends from the normal position of the meatus to the upper portion of the glans penis;
- penile epispadias, in which the opening involves the shaft and glans of the penis; and
- penopubic epispadias, in which the opening involves the entire length of the penis and a small area of the lower abdominal wall.

With the penopubic type of epispadias, eversion of part of the bladder through the opening may occur during coughing or straining.

b. In females. In females, the clitoris is bifid, and the open cleft extends along the length of the urethra up into the bladder neck. Incontinence is usually present. This defect is not as obvious in the female as in the male, and careful genital examination is necessary to detect it.

c. Treatment. Treatment of epispadias in the male requires surgery to reconstruct the urethra, straighten the penis, and restore continence. Mucosa and skin grafts are commonly used to close the urethra. Cosmetic surgery may be needed to create a normal-appearing penis. Extensive reconstructive surgery is necessary if exstrophy of the bladder is also present. Surgery for female epispadias involves excising skin and subcutaneous tissue and forming a tubular urethra of adequate length with an opening in the appropriate location.

Despite reconstruction, incontinence remains a major problem for children born with epispadias. Usually, some defect in the trigone or bladder neck coexists, and later surgery may be attempted to provide adequate bladder capacity and good muscle function as well as to correct vesicoureteric reflux, also commonly present. The success rate in achieving continence surgically is about 50 percent.

Nursing care must include having a knowledge of incontinence devices and teaching the child's parents to use them if necessary. A great deal of counseling is needed to aid the parents of the incontinent child to accept the situation and help the child to lead as normal a life as possible.

2. Hypospadias

Hypospadias is a common anomaly that occurs more frequently in male infants. The urethra fails to extend to the end of the penis, and the meatal opening is on the ventral side of the penile shaft. Hypospadias is classified according to location of the opening: glandular, penile, penile scrotal, and perineal (Figure 4-5).

a. Accompanying disorders. Anomalies commonly seen with hypospadias include bifid scrotum and cryptorchidism. Ventral curvature of the penis, or chordee, is almost always present. Other genitourinary anomalies may also be present.

Figure 4-5 *Hypospadias: A and B, penile; C and D, scrotal*

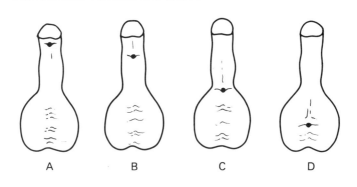

A B C D

b. Treatment. Surgical treatment involves reconstruction of the urethra, so that it extends to the glans penis, and correction of chordee. Circumcision should not be performed on these infants, as the foreskin will be needed for future surgery. Surgery is not done until the child is several years of age.

3. Posterior urethral valves

This anomaly is a common cause of urinary obstruction in males. Mucosal folds are present in the verumontanum (the area of the urethra where the ejaculatory ducts empty). These mucosal folds obstruct or prevent the flow of urine. The infant is born with dilated upper tracts, symptoms of azotemia, urinary tract infection, and possible obstructive uropathy leading to hyperkalemia. Some infants may not void at all. In this case, the damage to the upper tracts may be severe enough that ureteroileostomy or nephrostomy may be required to provide for adequate renal function. If the infant voids at all, transurethral resection of the valves may be all that is necessary to correct the disorder.

4. Other disorders of the urethra

a. Anterior urethral valves. This disorder is very rare. It involves the urethra above the membranous urethra and can be corrected transurethrally or by open surgery.

b. Meatal stenosis. There are varying degrees of stenosis. The upper urinary tract must be evaluated for possible damage. Meatotomy corrects the problem.

c. Urethrorectal fistulas. These fistulas usually occur in conjunction with imperforate anus.

F. Disorder of the testes: Cryptorchidism

Undescended testicles are very common in male infants. The cryptorchid testis failed to descend along its normal pathway or may be in the wrong position (Figure 4-6). This latter is more precisely called ectopic testis. In most cases, the undescended testicle can be located intra-abdominally in the inguinal canal or external ring. If it is ectopic, the testicle is usually at the base of the penis or in the opposite groin area. This condition may be bilateral or unilateral.

In many infants the testicle descends spontaneously. If, however, it has not descended by one year of age, hormonal therapy with human chorionic gonadotropin may cause the testicle to descend. If it does not, orchiopexy, or surgical placement of the testicle in its proper location in the scrotum, is done. The incidence of later development of testicular cancer is 40 times greater in the patient with cryptorchidism, even if spontaneous descent occurs. Parents should be made aware of this, so they can later have a health professional teach the young man the importance of testicular self-examination and how to do it.

Figure 4-6 *A, cryptorchidism; B, ectopic testis*

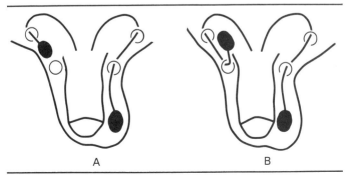

A

B

QUIZ

1. Ectopic kidneys can most often be located in the
   _____ .

2. In crossed renal ectopia, both kidneys are on the same
   side of the abdomen. They usually _____
   during fetal development.

3. In horseshoe kidney, the _____ poles of
   both kidneys fuse, and the fused kidney is located in
   the _____ .

4. The congenital, hereditary renal disease that develops
   later in life and involves the displacement of nephrons
   by cysts is called _____ .

5. Ureteropelvic junction obstruction is corrected surgically by a procedure called _____ .

6. Exstrophy of the bladder is usually accompanied by
   another anomaly, _____ of the urethra.

7. _____ is a possible major and lasting
   complication of epispadias, despite corrective surgery.

8. Abnormal location of the urinary opening on the
   ventral side of the penis is called _____ .

9. Posterior urethral valves are the most common cause
   of _____ in male infants.

10. Cryptorchidism is associated with a higher incidence
    of _____ in young men.

ANSWERS

1. Pelvis.
2. Fuse.
3. Lower, lower lumbar region.
4. Adult polycystic kidneys.
5. Pyeloplasty.

6. Epispadias.
7. Incontinence.
8. Hypospadias.
9. Urinary obstruction.
10. Testicular cancer.

C H A P T E R

Disorders of
the Kidney

OBJECTIVES

After completing this chapter, you will be able to:

1. *List the infectious, neoplastic, and traumatic disorders of the kidney, and tell how each is managed*

2. *Recognize the signs and symptoms of the various disorders of the kidney*

3. *Identify the diagnostic procedures used in the evaluation of the kidney*

4. *Understand nursing implications for a patient undergoing a nephrectomy*

5. *Understand the nursing implications for a patient with an infectious disorder of the kidney.*

A. Tumors

1. Benign tumors

Benign tumors of the kidney rarely present themselves as clinical problems because they usually do not develop enough to cause symptoms in the patient. The following are examples of such tumors:

- Lipomas are an aggregate of fat cells usually found in renal tissue. Usually they are so small that they do not produce symptoms.
- Myomas and leiomyomas are found under the renal capsule and are thought to originate from the capsule wall or from the blood vessel walls.
- Angiomyolipomas are small mesenchymal lesions usually found in the cortex or medulla of the kidney. They rarely become clinically significant.
- Cortical adenoma is significant because it is thought that renal cell carcinoma, a malignant tumor, originates from it because of their histologic similarity. The growth, which has a high lipid content, originates from tubular epithelium.

The benign tumors grow slowly and usually do not present symptoms, although there are cases in which the tumor has grown enough to cause pain. Renal function studies are normal, as are most intravenous pyelograms. A true diagnosis can only be made by an excision and biopsy of the mass. Symptomatic benign tumors are usually excised with conservation of the kidney.

2. Malignant tumors

Renal cell carcinoma (also known as adenocarcinoma and hypernephroma) accounts for approximately 80 percent of renal carcinomas. This tumor is usually found in people older than 50. After originating in the cortex, these tumors lie quiet for a long period. By the time symptoms appear, the tumor has usually extended through the renal capsule and into the pelvis.

a. Assessment. Hematuria, pain, and a renal mass are the "classic triad" of renal cancer. Although all these symptoms are found in only 15 percent of patients at the time of diagnosis, hematuria is present in 60 percent. Approximately 40 percent are discovered by accident. Fever and anemia may also be present. Usually, one or another of the symptoms of back pain, weight loss, and weakness causes the patient to seek medical advice.

These tumors metastasize most commonly to the lungs, brain, and bones by direct extension or via the vascular channels. The renal vein and vena cava are also common sites of metastasis. Twenty-five to 40 percent of patients present with metastases at time of diagnosis.

b. Diagnosis. A KUB (kidney-ureter-bladder) view, which outlines the borders of the kidney, is usually the first X-ray taken and may show a renal mass. An intravenous pyelogram will show some stretching and distortion of the calyces and also provide information from the normal kidney for purposes of comparison. Computed tomography (CT) is sometimes used to differentiate neoplasms from cysts.

After the preliminary X-rays are performed and it has been determined that a renal mass is present, a CT scan or ultrasound is performed. An ultrasound will differentiate a solid mass (tumor) from a fluid-filled mass (cyst). A needle biopsy of the kidney is usually not done if the mass is solid because of the danger of disseminating tumor cells that may be present.

A renal arteriogram can help to further evaluate the renal mass and its vascular outline. Arteriogram also helps in staging renal tumors by showing the presence of tumor in the renal vein or inferior vena cava.

Bone and liver scans are included in workups for metastatic cancer. A brain scan is indicated if there are signs of metastases.

c. Treatment. The treatment for renal cell cancer is radical nephrectomy, which includes excision of the perirenal fat and ureter. In many cases, a local para-aortic lymph node dissection is done to eliminate possible micrometastases. Embolization of kidney may be done preoperatively to reduce the vascularity of a large renal cancer.

Adjunctive X-ray or chemotherapy has not had satisfactory results in treating the primary tumor but may be used for metastases. The female hormone medroxyprogesterone (Depo-Provera) may be used for some patients postnephrectomy, though the rate of response to it is still under clinical investigation.

d. Nursing implications. During the pre-op period, explain to the patient the routine pre-op tests and other diagnostic studies he will receive. Potential for post-op complications can be reduced by adequate pre-op teaching of breathing exercises. Prior to surgery, the patient is shaved and prepped from nipple to mid-thigh on the side of the incision.

Provide emotional support and counseling for the patient and his family and allow the patient time to verbalize his feelings concerning his diagnosis of cancer.

The kidney is usually removed through a flank incision, a potential complication of which is pneumothorax. A chest X-ray is usually taken in the recovery room to evaluate the patient for any degree of pneumothorax.

Elastic stockings to provide venous support of the legs should be put on the patient during and after surgery. Post-op vital signs are usually taken every one to two hours for the first eight hours, then every two to four hours. Check the incisional flank dressings frequently for excessive bleeding.

The potential for respiratory complications can be reduced by maintaining a therapeutic respiratory regime and early mobilization.

B. Infectious disorders of the kidney

1. Pyelonephritis

Pyelonephritis is an infectious condition of the kidney that involves the renal parenchyma and collecting systems. The usual offending genera are *Proteus, Klebsiella, Pseudomonas, Staphylococcus* and coliform organisms, but any bacterium or fungus may cause the infection. In the majority of cases, the route of infection is from the lower urinary tract. Instrumentation and any obstructive uropathy are other causes of pyelonephritis.

a. Assessment. Assess your patient for these common symptoms of acute pyelonephritis: fever, chills, malaise, and urinary symptoms such as dysuria, urgency, and frequency. Hematuria may be present in some patients, as may nausea and vomiting. Diagnosis is made by a positive urine culture with a pathogen count of greater than 100,000 colonies per ml. the urine usually appears cloudy and is foul-smelling.

b. Treatment. Once appropriate cultures have been obtained, but before antibiotic therapy is started, any ureteral obstruction must be cleared. An obstructed kidney will not be able to concentrate antibiotics adequately. A urogram or cystogram may be done to detect an obstruction.

Hydration is important and an intravenous infusion may be started if the patient is unable to maintain an adequate fluid intake.

c. Nursing implications. During the acute phase of the infection the patient will have a need for pain relief. Analgesics are usually ordered for this reason. Bed rest may be prescribed, but usually for no more than five days. The patient is usually discharged on oral antimicrobial agents for a 10- to 14-day regimen. Discharge teaching should include the importance of completing the antibiotic regimen, the need for high fluid intake (unless contraindicated by another condition), and follow-up with routine cultures.

Avoidance of further infection is important for the prevention of chronic pyelonephritis, a progressive disease that results in scarring of the nephrons and, unless halted, can lead to renal failure.

2. Acute glomerulonephritis

Acute glomerulonephritis is an inflammatory condition of the glomerulus of the kidney caused by an antigen-antibody reaction. This disease usually occurs after a beta-hemolytic streptococcal infection elsewhere in the body (e.g., throat infection) for which the body produces antibody complexes. These antibodies collect in the glomerulus, causing inflammatory changes and decreased renal function. Glomerulonephritis is most frequently seen in children and teenagers.

a. Assessment and diagnosis. Onset of the disease is usually sudden. The patient may exhibit fever, chills, generalized edema, and other gastrointestinal symptoms such as nausea, vomiting, and/or anorexia. Gross hematuria and proteinuria due to the damaged basement membrane, are classic symptoms.

Because the kidneys are unable to concentrate urine, the specific gravity will be high, but urine output will be lower than normal. Serum BUN and creatinine levels may be elevated.

b. Treatment. Most patients recover from acute glomerular nephritis within two to three weeks. Treatment is supportive during this period. Bed rest may be recommended but has not been documented to affect the course of the disease. Dietary restrictions along with diuretic therapy may be prescribed for edema.

3. Renal carbuncle

A renal carbuncle is an abscess that is confined in the renal cortex, usually formed by penicillin-resistant staphylococcus. Hematogenous spread is thought to be the most common route of this infection, most likely from a skin lesion or the respiratory tract. Renal calculi and obstructive uropathy can also be sources of this infection.

Symptoms include fever, chills, and flank pain. Urine cultures may be negative since the abscess may not communicate with the collecting system. Diagnosis is made by intravenous pyelogram and or ultrasonography. A needle aspiration may be done to find out the culture and sensitivity of the organism. Intravenous antibiotic is usually the treatment of choice. Occasionally these abscesses require surgical drainage.

4. Perinephric abscess

A perinephric abscess is an infection of the fat-filled space around the kidney. It may be caused by nearby infection, such as a renal carbuncle, or by hematogenous spread of organisms from a distant infection.

Flank tenderness, fever, and chills are common symptoms. As with a renal carbuncle, intravenous pyelogram and ultrasonography are used in diagnosis. Treatment is usually surgical drainage in conjunction with antibiotic therapy. Sometimes nephrectomy is indicated.

5. Tuberculosis of the kidney

The kidney is rarely the primary site for tuberculosis. It is usually disseminated via the bloodstream from the lungs or gastrointestinal tract. The disease is usually present for a long time before symptoms appear, by which time much damage has already occurred to the kidney.

a. Course of the disease. The disease commonly affects both kidneys. It first affects the cortex and medulla, then progresses to the renal pelvis. From the pelvis, the disease can spread to other areas of the genitourinary system. Cystitis and/or epididymitis in males are usually the earliest symptoms. Other symptoms include frequency and burning with urination.

b. Diagnosis. Diagnosis is made by urine culture. Usually early-morning specimens taken on three to six days are needed to make the diagnosis, since the tubercle bacilli are shed intermittently.

c. Treatment. Treatment includes combination chemotherapy for a minimum of two years. Isoniazid (INH), ethambutol (Myambutol) and rifampin (Rifadin) are drugs frequently used together. Nephrectomy is indicated with the failure of chemotherapy. Followup is important with these patients, and compliance with the chemotherapy regimen is necessary for successful treatment.

C. Trauma

Although the kidney is well protected by a tough fibrous capsule and other body structures (rib cage and back muscles), it can nonetheless undergo trauma. Traffic accidents, falls, and contact-sports injuries, especially from football, are the major causes for nonpenetrating renal trauma. Gunshot wounds and stabbings account for a large percentage of the penetrating injuries.

1. Types of injuries

Injuries to the kidney may be classified into four groups: contusions, lacerations, fractures, and injuries to the renal pedicle.

a. Contusions or subcapsular hematomas. These account for 70 to 80 percent of all renal injuries. Minor cortical lacerations are also classified under contusions. These injuries usually do not involve the renal collecting system, and most are considered relatively minor. Symptoms are unremarkable, though some patients complain of intermittent hematuria and flank pain. Treatment is conservative, and healing usually occurs spontaneously.

b. Lacerations. A tear may extend into the renal parenchyma and cause a hematoma in the renal pelvis. Injuries of this nature are more serious and may require surgical intervention to repair the tear or drain the hematoma. Patients require close watching for symptoms of hemorrhage. Hemoglobin and hematocrit values must be monitored for any decrease. Vital signs are to be checked frequently.

c. Fracture. A kidney fracture occurs when the renal tissue or parenchyma is shattered. Damage to the kidney is extensive and usually involves the collecting system. Often an immediate nephrectomy must be performed to prevent hemorrhage.

d. Damage to the renal pedicle. The renal pedicle holds the renal artery and other important circulatory and nervous system connections for the kidney, and injury to it is very serious. Usually the kidney cannot be salvaged, especially if the kidney has no collateral circulation. This type of injury can be life-threatening, and treatment must be prompt.

2. Assessment and diagnosis

Since renal trauma is usually associated with other injuries, an overall assessment must be made. Along with urinalysis, urine should also be tested for microscopic hematuria. Renal function studies are also done. An intravenous urogram may show delayed function, incomplete filling, and extravasation in or outside of the renal capsule. Renal arteriograms are helpful in the diagnosis and visualization of damage to the kidney's vascular tree.

QUIZ

1. One difference between a renal cyst and a renal tumor is that on X-ray examination a cyst appears (and is) _____ and a tumor has a _____ appearance.

2. _____, _____, _____, are the classic triad of symptoms for renal cell carcinoma.

3. A _____ X-ray is generally the first taken to evaluate the kidney. It is followed by a (n) _____.

4. Urine of patients with pyelonephritis usually appears _____ and is _____.

5. _____ and _____ are classic symptoms of glomerulonephritis.

6. _____, _____, and _____ are major causes of nonpenetrating renal trauma.

7. Renal trauma can be classified in four categories: _____, _____, _____, and _____.

ANSWERS

1. Fluid-filled, solid.
2. Hematuria, pain, renal mass.
3. KUB (kidneys-ureter-bladder), IVP (intravenous pyelogram).
4. Cloudy, foul-smelling.
5. Gross hematuria, proteinuria.
6. Traffic accidents, falls, and contact sports.
7. Contusions, lacerations, fractures, pedicle injuries.

6

Disorders of the Bladder

OBJECTIVES

After completing this chapter, you will be able to:

1. *Describe the common causes, diagnosis, and treatment of urinary tract infections*

2. *List the several anatomic disorders of the bladder, their symptomatology, and the surgical procedures used to correct them*

3. *Describe the etiology of neurogenic bladder dysfunction and its resulting symptoms and treatments*

4. *Aid the patient with cancer of the bladder to understand the diagnostic tests and surgeries used in evaluation and treatment*

5. *Provide the bladder cancer patient with information and counseling to promote as normal a lifestyle as possible.*

Introduction

1. Symptoms

Many bladder disorders share similar symptomatology. Patients with infectious, anatomic, and neurogenic disorders experience varying degrees of symptoms, including frequency, urgency, nocturia, dysuria, and, possibly, incontinence. All of these symptoms are most distressing to patients who find that their lives begin to revolve around necessary proximity to a toilet.

The exceptions to this are the neoplastic disorders. Painless hematuria is a heralding symptom of carcinoma with an origin somewhere in the urinary tract. Some patients simply notice the presence of blood in urine. Other patients may be informed, after urinalysis done for routine reasons, that there are traces of blood in their urine. Hematuria is not absolutely diagnostic of cancer, so it is essential that all patients with hematuria undergo intravenous pyelogram and cystoscopy to rule out carcinoma.

2. Diagnostic tests

Many radiologic tests help the physician to identify the cause of a patient's symptoms. Urodynamic studies, which evaluate lower urinary tract disorders, are commonly used. These studies will be discussed along with the disorders.

Infectious disorders

A. Cystitis

Cystitis, or urinary tract infection (UTI), is common among women. It is characterized by frequency, suprapubic pain, urgency, dysuria, and, occasionally, hematuria.

1. Etiology

a. In women. Cystitis is easy for women to acquire due to the shorter length of the urethra and its proximity to the vagina and rectum, both of which are normally abundant with flora. Poor perineal hygiene, sexual intercourse, and use of the diaphragm have all been associated with cystitis.

b. In men. Cystitis in men may result from obstructive lower urinary tract disorders such as prostatism or urethral strictures. Inability to completely empty the bladder leads to increasing amounts of residual urine. Stasis of urine in the bladder causes normally harmless bacteria to multiply and cause cystitis. This is true also for women who are unable to empty their bladders.

2. Diagnosis

Cystitis is diagnosed by history, physical examination, urinalysis, and urine culture. Specimens should be obtained by clean-catch midstream or catheterization. Urinalysis reveals bacteria and white blood cells in the urine. Urine culture isolates and identifies the causative organism and its antimicrobial sensitivities.

3. Prevention and treatment

a. Uncomplicated UTI. For simple, uncomplicated cystitis, a course of appropriate oral antibiotics will cure the infection. Table 6-1 lists the antibiotics that physicians most commonly prescribe. Bladder analgesics such as phenazopyridine help to alleviate symptoms during the initial days of antibiotic therapy.

TABLE 6-1
COMMON URINARY TRACT ANTIBIOTICS

Ampicillin
Cephalexin (Keflex)
Cephradine (Velosef)
Nitrofurantoin (Macrodantin)
Sulfisoxazole (Gantrisin)
Tetracycline
Trimethoprim/Sulfamethoxazole (Bactrim, Septra)

b. Complicated UTI. Patients with recurrent or complicated UTIs must undergo further workup. Urologists look for anatomic abnormalities that may interfere with normal voiding and predispose the patient to infection. Common tests include intravenous pyelogram, cystoscopy, urethroscopy, cystogram, voiding cystourethrogram, and urodynamics. If no abnormality is found, the patient may be placed on a prophylactic dose of a urinary tract antibiotic in an attempt to keep him or her infection-free. If an anatomic abnormality is present, its correction is usually all that is needed to restore sterile urine.

c. Treatment. Urethral dilation with metal sounds has been a common practice for treating women with recurrent UTI. The theory is that scar tissue buildup from previous infections interferes with voiding. Dilation is intended to stretch the urethra. This practice has fallen out of favor, as urologists recognize that this painful procedure does not significantly reduce infection.

Urethral strictures or stenosis is very rare in women. It is not unusual, however, for some urologists to recommend urethral reconstruction (urethroplasty) or surgical enlargement of the meatus (meatotomy) to decrease the rate of infection in female patients.

d. Catheter-related UTIs. It has long been recognized that indwelling Foley catheters are the leading cause of nosocomial infections and UTIs in hospitalized patients. As many as 90 percent with Foley catheters may develop UTI within five days. Infectious-disease specialists and urologists recommend the use of Foley catheters only when absolutely necessary.

B. Interstitial cystitis

1. Diagnosis

Interstitial cystitis is characterized by severe discomfort when voiding, decreased bladder capacity, and extreme frequency and urgency. Its etiology is unknown. Interstitial cystitis is diagnosed by cystoscopy and bladder biopsies that reveal fibrosis, inflammation, and edema of the bladder wall. The fibrotic process of this disease causes the bladder wall to stiffen and lose its ability to store increasing amounts of urine. Urine cultures are usually negative.

2. Treatment

The most frequently used treatment for interstitial cystitis is treatments with DMSO (dimethyl sulfoxide), usually done in the doctor's office. DMSO is instilled into the bladder through a catheter and retained for a period, then voided out. Some urologists add steroids to the DMSO to decrease its irritating effects. Results are usually dramatic, with a marked improvement in symptoms after several treatments.

Other forms of cystitis

Tuberculosis, radiation treatments, trauma, schistosomiasis, and uremia can all lead to various forms of cystitis. These are special cases, usually diagnosed by pathologic examinations of biopsies and X-ray studies. Treatment depends on the causative disease.

Anatomic disorders of the bladder

The most severe anatomic abnormalities of the bladder are congenital. A variety of conditions, however, may cause bladder symptomatology. These are described here.

Trauma (perforation of the bladder)

Injury to the pelvic area in accidents, resulting in fractured pelvis, or crushing or penetrating wounds may cause bladder perforation. Surgical perforation may occur accidentally during instrumentation with catheters, sounds, or cystoscopes or during transurethral resections of prostate or bladder tumors. The patient experiences pain, the pelvis is dull to percussion, and the abdomen is rigid. Diagnosis is confirmed by X-ray when contrast material injected into the bladder urethrally is seen outside the bladder. Treatment is surgical closure of the bladder with possible temporary suprapubic cystotomy.

Diverticuli

A bladder diverticulum is a herniation of the bladder mucosa through the bladder's muscular wall. It can be the result of continuous attempts to void when significant urethral resistance is present (as in prostatic hypertrophy). Small diverticuli that empty completely during voiding usually don't cause a problem. Small or large diverticuli that do not empty may lead to recurrent infections. Some diverticuli can grow to be larger than the bladder itself. In severe cases, surgical repair is necessary.

C. Bladder decompensation: Hyporeflexia

Bladder decompensation can also result from voiding against increased urethral resistance. It occurs as the detrusor muscle gradually loses its ability to contract (hyporeflexia). The result of this can range from increasing amounts of residual urine to total urinary retention. Since this is a gradual process, retention is usually not painful, despite large amounts of urine in the bladder. The patient may carry over 1000 cc of urine in the bladder even after voiding.

1. Diagnosis

Diagnosis is made by measuring residual urine, which can be done by catheterization, or by estimating it during X-ray studies. Urodynamic studies also help to diagnose hyporeflexia. In severe cases, urine may back up into the ureters, leading to hydronephrosis and pyelonephritis. Chronically overdistended bladders are also more susceptible to infection.

2. Treatment

Treatment is primarily removal of the cause of increased urethral resistance or obstruction. Afterward, intermittent catheterization may be necessary temporarily or permanently. Patients facing permanent lack of bladder function and self-catheterization will require much reassurance and explanation from you. No medication will satisfactorily restore bladder function. You must ascertain from the physician the probability of restored bladder function before offering the patient any hope that the situation is temporary.

D. Bladder decompensation: Hyperreflexia

The opposite of hyporeflexia, this type of bladder decompensation results in a spastic bladder with a decreased capacity, one that simply contracts without the patient's volition. The result of this ranges from urgency to incontinence. Increased urethral resistance is also among the causative factors of hyperreflexia.

1. Diagnosis

History and urologic tests, including urodynamics and voiding cystourethrograms, aid in diagnosis. With significant obstruction, the patient's flow may be poor, despite the strong involuntary bladder contraction. Removal of the cause of obstruction may result in a gradual return to normal bladder function, while in some patients the hyperreflexia persists.

2. Treatment

Treatment of hyperreflexia due to obstruction is similar to treatment of hyperreflexia of neurogenic origin and is covered in the section on neurogenic bladder dysfunction.

Stress incontinence

1. Description

Stress incontinence is most often the result of pelvic floor relaxation in females following childbirth or pelvic surgery. The bladder and urethra descend into the weakened vaginal wall, possibly creating a cystocele and urethrocele. The cystocele may be quite obvious when observing the external genitalia, appearing as a bulge below the meatus. Stress incontinence may be present without a cystocele and/or urethrocele.

The patient with stress incontinence leaks urine when abdominal pressure is increased – for example, when coughing, laughing, jumping, straining, or valsalva. In severe cases, leakage may occur when the patient rises from a supine to a standing position. Constant dribbling during exercise, even walking, may also occur.

2. Diagnosis

Diagnosis is made by cystoscopy and urethroscopy, voiding cystourethrogram, and urodynamics. If the degree of stress incontinence is not severe, conservative treatment with medi-

TABLE 6-2

MEDICATIONS USED IN BLADDER DISORDERS

To decrease detrusor hyperreflexia
Anticholinergics   Propantheline (Pro-Banthine)   Tincture of belladonna (used only for children)   *Antidepressants*   Impiramine HCl (Tofranil)   *Antispasmodics*   Baclofen (Lioresal)   Dicyclomine HCl (Bentyl)   Oxybutynin Cl (Ditropan)
To increase outlet resistance
Ephedrine   Phenylpropanolamine HCl   Pseudoephedrine HCl
To decrease outlet resistance
Prazosin HCl (Minipress)

cation may restore the patient to a satisfactory state of "dryness" (see Table 6-2).

3. Treatment

Surgery for correction of stress incontinence follows all of the testing already mentioned as well as discussion between the patient and the urologist to determine how much the condition bothers the patient. If the patient would rather live with the condition than undergo surgery to correct it, her wishes should be respected. If the condition is extremely distressing to the patient, she may welcome the idea of corrective surgery. The most common procedures to correct stress incontinence are outlined below.

a. Vaginal repair (anterior colporrhaphy). An incision is made into the anterior vaginal wall, vaginal hysterectomy is performed, and sutures are placed on either side of the bladder neck to restore the normal angle of the urethra and bladder. For several days post-op, the patient will have an indwelling Foley catheter.

b. Endoscopic bladder neck suspension (Stamey procedure). Two suprapubic incisions are made on either side of midline, and an anterior vaginal wall incision is also made. Needles are passed through the suprapubic incisions, through the rectus muscle, and guided downward lateral to the bladder neck and into the vaginal incision. Suture material is passed through the needles, and, when tightened, they elevate the bladder neck to its proper position. Cystoscopes are used during the procedure to make sure that the needles have not passed through the bladder wall.

Postoperatively, the patient will have an indwelling suprapubic tube, which is clamped on approximately the third post-op day. The tube is removed when the patient is able to void well.

c. Suprapubic procedures. Through a vertical suprapubic incision, the bladder is separated from the vagina, and sutures are placed into the area of the proximal urethra and bladder neck. These sutures are then anchored into the pubic bone. In some cases, the urethra is lengthened with a piece of urethrovesical wall.

After surgery, the vagina is packed with gauze until the patient is fully awake, and an indwelling catheter is left in place for one day.

d. Pubovaginal sling. This operation is most often performed on patients who have failed one or more of the above surgeries for stress incontinence.The surgeon creates a sling from the patient's rectal fascia and places it across the urethra, obstructing the nonfunctional area that is causing the incontinence.

Postoperatively, patients will have a Foley catheter or suprapubic tube for five to seven days. The majority of these patients will need to self-catheterize after the operation, possibly always.

All patients undergoing surgery for stress incontinence should be treated with antibiotics postoperatively. A patient who has trouble voiding after the operation may need to learn intermittent self-catheterization until normal voiding function returns.

F. Post-prostatectomy incontinence

Total or partial incontinence is a potential complication of prostatectomy. This occurs more frequently in patients who have undergone transurethral prostate resection. There are several causes for this incontinence.

1. Preoperative hyperreflexia

Patients with demonstrated hyperreflexia before surgery are likely to have some degree of urgency incontinence postoperatively. After removal of the obstructing prostate, the involuntary contractions of the bladder simply propel urine out the urethra. Some patients can control this with contraction of the sphincter muscles, and others cannot. This condition may or may not subside.

Figure 6-1 *Artificial urethral sphincter;* courtesy American Medical Systems Inc., Minnetonka, Minn.

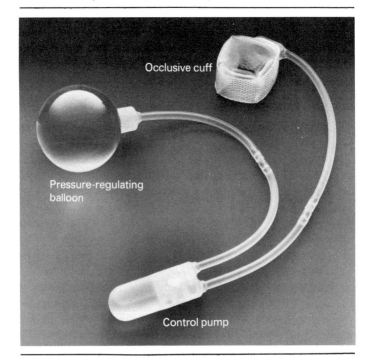

2. Stress incontinence

Rigorous resection of the prostate may result in damage to the bladder neck, leaving the patient unable to control the flow of urine when abdominal pressure is increased, especially when the bladder is full. Some degree of urgency incontinence may also be present: The patient begins to leak urine when he experiences the urge to void, before he can get to a toilet.

3. Total incontinence

Complete urinary incontinence results from damage to both the bladder neck and the voluntary sphincter musculature. The bladder is simply unable to retain any urine, and contrast urinary leakage occurs.

4. Treatment

There are various treatments for post-prostatectomy incontinence. Medication may improve the situation for some patients (see Table 6-2). Electrical stimulation has helped to increase pelvic floor muscle control and decrease incontinence. If the patient is totally incontinent, he will have to wear an external collecting device. Foley catheters are recommended only for patients who cannot be fitted with an external collecting device.

Improvements in the design of an artificial urethral sphincter have provided an alternative for this group of patients (Figure 6-1). A fluid-filled cuff is surgically placed around the urethra near the bladder neck. The cuff is connected to a fluid reservoir, which is placed under the rectus muscle, and an activating pump is placed in the scrotum (or the labia in females). Squeezing the pump deflates the cuff, and the patient's bladder is drained of urine. At all other times, the cuff is inflated, compressing the urethra and keeping the patient continent.

G. Bladder neck contracture

Contracture of the bladder neck creates symptoms similar to prostatism: decreased stream, frequency, nocturia, and incomplete bladder emptying. The cause may be congenital or acquired as a result of fibrosis, probably secondary to inflammation. Bladder neck contracture is frequently a complication of transurethral resection of the prostate.

Diagnosis is made by cystoscopy, voiding cystourethrogram, and urodynamics. Surgical correction is by transurethral incision of the bladder neck or, less frequently, suprapubic bladder neck revision. Both of these procedures may result in incontinence – particularly in females – and, possibly, retrograde ejaculation in males.

H. Vesicovaginal fistula

Occasionally a complication of abdominal hysterectomy, other pelvic surgery, or a complicated obstetrical delivery, formation of a vesicovaginal fistula results in constant and continuous urine leakage. Small amounts of urine may be retained in the vagina by contraction of the pelvic floor muscles. In some cases, the patient leaks only during stress.

1. Diagnosis

Diagnosis is made by cystoscopy. Some physicians instill methylene blue into the bladder through a catheter and observe for vaginal leakage. Most patients must wait 10 to 12 weeks after the causative surgery or injury before undergoing surgical repair of the fistula. An indwelling Foley catheter can keep the patient dry.

2. Treatment

Repair of the fistula is performed either transvaginally or transvesically. The transvaginal approach involves excision of the fistulous tract and closure of the bladder wall and vagina. If the repair is done transvesically, the fistula is excised via an incision into the bladder. The vaginal wall is closed, as is the area of the bladder wall where the fistula opened, and then the bladder itself.

Postoperatively, the bladder is drained by a suprapubic catheter to prevent urinary leakage to the incision line. The vagina may be packed with gauze for the first 24 hours. After one to two weeks, a cystogram is performed to check for leakage. If there is no leakage, the catheter is removed.

Neurogenic bladder dysfunction

A. Background

1. Dysfunctional state

It has long been accepted that the sacral spinal cord is the reflex neurologic center for voiding, particularly segments S_2 to S_4. Research has shown that areas of the brain are also involved in the initiation of the voiding reflex. Therefore, injury or disease of the sacral spinal cord or the brain, as well as any area of the nervous system in between, can result in some degree of voiding dysfunction (Figure 6-2).

Figure 6-2 *Neurologic pathways of voiding reflex;* from Greene LF, Segura JW, eds: *Transurethral Surgery.* Philadelphia: Saunders, 1979.

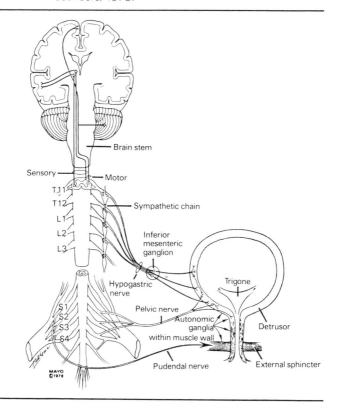

Most of these disorders involve either an inability to empty the bladder or an inability to store urine in the bladder. Drug therapy, intermittent self-catheterization, and simple surgical procedures can be used singly or in combination to help the patient achieve satisfactory bladder function.

2. Normal bladder emptying

Normally, the bladder can accommodate increasing amounts of urine at a low intravesical pressure. As the bladder fills — up to 400 cc — stretch receptors in the bladder wall are stimulated, creating the urge to void. If a toilet is not available, a person can inhibit voiding, despite a full bladder and an urge to void, by voluntarily contracting the pelvic floor and sphincter muscles. There should not be any involuntary leakage of urine. When he or she reaches an appropriate place to void, neurologic messages are sent from the brain down the spinal cord to the sacral cord area, causing the bladder's detrusor muscle to contract, intravesical pressure to rise sharply, and pelvic floor muscles and sphincter muscles to relax as voiding occurs.

Normally, a person nearly completely empties his or her bladder when voiding. Residual urine volumes greater than 100 cc are considered abnormal.

3. Viewpoint

We look at neurogenic bladder dysfunction in this chapter according to the symptoms exhibited by the patient. A few of the many neurologic disorders that cause these symptoms are outlined, and current methods of treatment are introduced. Keep in mind that treatment of such disorders is constantly changing. It is not at all unlikely that you will encounter a totally unfamiliar treatment or surgical intervention in the course of your work.

B. Detrusor hyperreflexia

Detrusor hyperreflexia is a common neurologic disorder of the bladder. The symptoms are the same as those described under hyperreflexia due to bladder decompensation. Unlike bladder decompensation, however, sensation may or may not be present, and there usually is no obstruction. This type of hyperreflexia is the result of some neurologic defect that affects the brain or sacral spinal cord tract.

1. Diagnosis

Urodynamics aids in diagnosis. Cystoscopy and radiographic studies rule out anatomic disorders, urine cultures rule out infection. Detrusor hyperreflexia is seen when the disorder or defect is above the level of the sacral voiding center. Among the causes are spinal cord injury or tumors, multiple sclerosis, Parkinson's disease, vertebral disc disorders, and cerebrovascular accident. This type of bladder dysfunction is also called spastic, uninhibited, or upper motor neuron neurogenic bladder.

2. Treatment

a. Medications. Treatment usually involves anticholinergic and antispasmodic drugs. Antidepressant medication in small doses may accentuate these other medications. Depending on the severity of the condition, pharmacologic treatment may help to reduce or prevent the uninhibited contractions. In some patients, the drugs work so well that complete retention results, and the patient must perform self-catheterization. For many patients, particularly those without bladder sensation, this is far preferable to incontinence. Table 6-2 lists drugs commonly used to treat hyperreflexia.

b. Surgery. Surgical intervention may be considered if medications have failed. Several procedures are used, the most common of which are bladder denervation, which involves incising the bladder wall and attempting to sever nerve supply to the bladder; and augmentation cystoplasty, which enlarges the size of the bladder by surgically adding a section of bowel. Either of these operations, if successful, results in complete retention, and the patient must learn self-catheterization.

3. Patient teaching

You have several responsibilities when caring for the patient with detrusor hyperreflexia. It's likely that you'll have to teach self-catheterization, a task that requires patience and considerable practice. You can help prepare the patient for therapy by explaining the side effects of anticholinergic medications. Most importantly, assume an attitude that communicates understanding of the underlying disorder and that does not make the patient feel guilty about his or her lack of bladder control.

C. Detrusor areflexia

Detrusor areflexia, also called flaccid hyporeflexia or lower motor neuron neurogenic bladder, results from neurologic injury to the sacral spinal cord, cauda equina, or sacral roots or nerves. In some cases, sensation may be present, though usually it isn't. The bladder fills continuously with urine until it reaches capacity, at which point overflow incontinence may occur. Among the causes of this type of bladder dysfunction are diabetes mellitus, tabes dorsalis, spinal cord injury or tumor, and disc disorders. Left untreated, areflexia can lead to upper tract changes such as hydronephrosis, ultimately compromising renal function.

1. Diagnosis

Urodynamic studies reveal a large-capacity bladder, usually with low intravesical filling pressure. Voluntary or involuntary contractions are absent. The patient is unable to void. Radiographic studies are done to evaluate the upper tract. Cystoscopy rules out obstructive or anatomic causes.

2. Treatment

Treatment involves regimens of Crede maneuver, abdominal straining, initiation of reflex contractions (if possible) or self-catheterization. Crede maneuver involves applying pressure to the suprapubic area to overcome resistance and force urine out of the bladder. Abdominal straining requires strong abdominal muscle control. The patient "bears down" to force urine out. Reflex contractions may be initiated by manually stimulating such areas as the glans penis, clitoris, or pubic hair. None of these is considered successful if there is excess residual urine. Intermittent catheterization is the treatment of choice if the patient or a family member is able to perform it. Otherwise, indwelling Foley catheters or supra-pubic tubes are a last resort. At present, there are no known medications that can restore bladder function.

D. Detrusor-sphincter dyssynergia

Detrusor-sphincter dyssynergia is a neurologic condition in which the striated or smooth sphincter musculature contracts at the same time as a voluntary or involuntary bladder contraction. Voiding is difficult for patients with dyssynergia, as the involuntary contraction of the sphincter muscle obstructs the flow of urine. This disorder is seen almost only in patients with spinal cord injury.

1. Diagnosis and treatment

Extensive and sophisticated urodynamic and radiographic studies are required to diagnose this condition. Treatment involves transurethral surgical incision of the sphincter muscle to prevent contraction.

2. Incontinence

If the patient has hyperreflexia along with the dyssynergia, he or she will be incontinent after the surgery. This is clinically preferable to dyssynergia, which can lead to upper tract deterioration. Anticholinergic medications, self-catheterization, or external collecting devices can be used to manage the resulting incontinence.

Neoplastic disorders

A. Background

1. Incidence

Cancer of the bladder is the most common of all urinary tract carcinomas. It is estimated that this disease caused 10,600 deaths in the United States in 1982. Its peak incidence occurs in the 50- to 70-year-old age group, with men affected two to three times more frequently than women. Ninety-seven percent of all bladder tumors are of epithelial origin, and of those, 90 percent are transitional cell tumors.

2. Etiology

Many factors have been linked to the development of bladder cancer, including cigarette smoking, industrial exposure to chemicals found in the textile and rubber industries, artificial sweeteners (saccharin), coffee, analgesics (phenacetin), and pelvic irradiation. Chronic irritation by indwelling catheters may lead to bladder cancer, as may bladder diverticuli. Urinary schistosomiasis has been linked to squamous cell carcinoma of the bladder.

B. Signs and symptoms

The heralding sign of bladder cancer is hematuria, which is present in three-fourths of all cases. The hematuria may be microscopic or "silent" (detectable only by urinalysis) or it may be gross (clearly visible in the urine). As tumor growth spreads, bladder symptoms may be experienced: frequency, dysuria, urgency, and suprapubic discomfort. Urinary tract infection may also occur. For this reason, treatment and evaluation of recurrent UTI must include intravenous pyelogram and cystoscopy to rule out bladder tumor.

Symptoms may not occur until the cancer is invasive, extending into the bladder wall. Early transitional cell tumors are papillary, resembling small outpouches inside the bladder. These are usually asymptomatic. Many patients experience no symptoms until metastasis.

C. Diagnosis

1. Visualizations

Cystoscopy is the first step in diagnosing bladder cancer. Both invasive and papillary tumors are easily seen through a cystoscope. Intravenous pyelogram may show a filling defect in the bladder wall, which may or may not represent a bladder tumor. Cytologic examinations of urine specimens may disclose atypical or malignant cells in the urine. Examined specimens are evaluated from Class 0 to Class 5. Class 0 is normal; Class 5 is absolutely diagnostic of carcinoma somewhere in the urinary tract.

2. Tissue biopsy

Biopsies of the bladder wall are usually taken at the same time cystoscopy is done. Tissue is taken from the affected areas and examined to determine the extent of invasion into the bladder wall. The pathologist assigns a stage to the specimens taken. Based on the findings, further testing, treatment, and, if necessary, surgical intervention is planned.

The following is the most commonly used staging system for bladder cancer (see Figure 6-3):
- Stage 0: Tumor confined to the mucosa
- Stage A: No tumor penetration beneath the lamina propria (the layer of connective and elastic tissue between the inner mucosa and detrusor muscle layer)
- Stage B_1: Tumor has extended into but not more than halfway through the muscle layer
- Stage B_2: Tumor has extended more than halfway through the muscle layer, but does not invade the perivesical tissue
- Stage C: Tumor has penetrated into the perivesical connective tissue
- Stage D_1: Metastatic disease to the pelvis, particularly the pelvic lymph nodes
- Stage D_2: Metastatic disease outside the pelvis.

Figure 6-3 *Staging classification of bladder cancer*

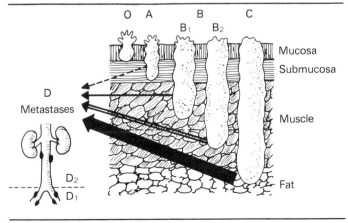

D. Further evaluation and treatment

The patient diagnosed as having bladder cancer may need to undergo many additional tests as part of a metastatic evaluation. The extent of further testing depends upon the results of the tests already done, especially the disease stage determined by the pathologist after biopsy.

1. Early-stage tumors

a. Surgical resection. For patients with Stage 0 bladder tumors, surgical resection is performed transurethrally, with instruments passed through a cystoscope. If only a single or just a few tumors are present, this may be the only necessary treatment. If many tumors are found or if there is a concentration of tumors in one area of the bladder, other approaches may be used.

b. Chemotherapy. Intravenous chemotherapy has proven helpful in decreasing the recurrence of these papillary tumors. Thiotepa and mitomycin-C (Mutamycin) are the currently used chemotherapeutic agents. The drug is introduced into the bladder through a catheter, retained by the patient for a specified period, then voided out. The frequency of these treatments is decided by the physician.

c. Partial cystectomy. If many tumors are confined to one area, partial cystectomy may be performed. This surgical procedure involves opening the bladder wall through a suprapubic incision and excising the affected area. The bladder wall is then resutured together. Suprapubic and Foley catheter drainage is maintained for several days postoperatively. Following removal of the drainage catheters, patients notice a dramatic reduction in bladder capacity, which gradually increases as healing occurs.

d. Follow-up. Close follow-up is extremely important for these patients, as 70 percent of superficial or papillary bladder tumors recur at some time. Patients *must* have periodic cystoscopies to watch for recurrence. The frequency of these cystoscopies decreases as the time since the last recurrence or original occurrence increases.

TABLE 6-3

TESTS TO EVALUATE FOR METASTATIC BLADDER CANCER

Test	Purpose
Random bladder biopsies	To rule out carcinoma in situ where papillary tumors are not obvious.
Bimanual exam under anesthesia	To evaluate extent of pelvic fixation, which occurs with spread of disease outside the bladder.
Chest X-ray and/or tomography	To rule out metastases to the lungs.
Intravenous pyelogram	To look for ureteral obstruction or deviation secondary to spread of disease around the bladder or to the pelvic lymph nodes.
Routine blood chemistry studies	To rule out azotemia and evaluate liver function.
Bone scan	To look for bone metastases. Lesions found are usually biopsied.
CAT scan	To look for enlarged lymph nodes in the pelvis and for perivesical involvement. Enlarged lymph nodes are also usually biopsied.
Urinary cytology	To detect atypical or malignant cells in the urine.
Liver scan	To detect liver metastases.
Pelvic lymphadenectomy	A surgical procedure, usually done at the time of cystectomy and diversion, to define extent of disease spread to the pelvic lymph nodes.

e. Stage A and Stage B₁. Stage B_1 bladder tumors are treated similarly to Stage 0. In some cases, cystectomy and diversion may be necessary. Usually, these patients undergo more frequent intravesical chemotherapy treatments.

2. Late-stage tumors

1. Stage B₂ and Stage C. Patients with Stages B_2 or C bladder cancer undergo radical surgery. Evaluation for metastases precedes surgery and includes tests that search for metastases to pelvic and periaortic lymph nodes, lung, liver, and bone. Table 6-3 outlines the tests involved in the metastatic evaluation. It is obvious by the number and type of tests that the stage of disease assigned to the patient may be changed by the results of these tests.

b. Stage B$_2$, Stage C, and Stage D. Stages B$_2$, C, and D bladder cancer patients may undergo radiation treatments prior to surgery. Radical surgery includes removal of the bladder (cystectomy), creation of a urinary stoma or urostomy with a section of ileum and pelvic lymphadenectomy. In females, the entire urethra, anterior vaginal wall, uterus, cervix, fallopian tubes, and ovaries are also removed. In males, the prostate, seminal vesicles, and proximal urethra are removed.

c. Widespread disease. If extensive metastatic disease is present, surgery may or may not be performed. Systemic chemotherapy using cisplatin (Platinol), cyclophosphamide (Cytoxan), and doxorubicin (Adriamycin) can be used. Postoperative radiation therapy may be used, or radiation therapy and systemic chemotherapy in combination with or without surgery.

E. Implications for the patient with bladder cancer

1. Life-style changes

Even patients with Stage 0 disease experience a dramatic change in life-style following diagnosis. Follow-up cystoscopies are required for the remainder of their lives.

Patients with disease requiring radical surgery face change in body image and, especially for men, almost certain loss of sexual ability. They must learn to adapt to their urinary stoma and appearance. They must also face lifelong follow-up. Postoperative cystectomy and diversion patients must have periodic intravenous pyelograms, as transitional cell carcinoma may recur in the ureters or renal pelvis. Men must also have periodic urethroscopies.

2. Complications of surgery

As with all radical surgeries, early and late complications can occur. Early complications include those common to most major surgeries, as well as wound infection, wound dehiscence, ureteral leaks, sepsis, and azotemia (possibly leading to renal insufficiency and failure). Late complications include stomal stenosis, stricture formation or obstruction at the ureteroileal anastomosis (leading to hydronephrosis and azotemia), stone formation, chronic urinary tract infection, hyperchloremic acidosis, intestinal obstruction, parastomal hernias, and uremia.

3. Nursing implications

Nursing care of the patient who is being evaluated for metastatic disease or who has undergone cystectomy and diversion is extensive and important. It is your responsibility to help the patient and his or her family to manage the urostomy. If at all possible, an enterostomal therapist should be consulted. The therapist marks a stoma site on the patient's abdomen preoperatively and selects an appliance postoperatively that the patient can most easily manage and obtain. Numerous appliances are now available.

The ability of the urostomy patient to return to a normal life-style depends on the information and teaching provided during the period of hospitalization and immediately after discharge. Nurses play a major role in this period of crisis by sharing knowledge and coordinating available services to help the patient's physical and emotional recovery.

QUIZ

1. Symptoms of cystitis include _____,
_____, _____,
and _____.

2. Trauma to the bladder commonly results from
_____.

3. Hyporeflexia bladder usually results in _____
of urine.

4. Hyperreflexic bladder is characterized by _____ _____ contractions of the bladder muscle.

5. Leakage of urine during increased abdominal pressure in females is called _____.

6. Incontinence after transurethral surgery of the prostate can be of three types: _____, _____, or _____.

7. A common complication of hysterectomy, pelvic surgery, or complicated obstetrical delivery is _____.

8. Treatment of neurogenic detrusor hyperreflexia may include three classes of drugs: _____, _____, _____.

9. Patients with detrusor areflexia frequently need to learn _____.

10. Stage 0 carcinoma of the bladder is treated by _____ and follow-up periodic _____.

ANSWERS

1. Frequency, suprapubic pain, urgency, dysuria.
2. Accidental injury to the pelvis.
3. Retention.
4. Involuntary.
5. Stress incontinence.
6. Hyperreflexic (urge), stress, total.
7. Vesicovaginal fistula.
8. Anticholinergics, antispasmodics, antidepressants.
9. Intermittent self-catheterization.
10. Transurethral resection of bladder tumors, cystoscopies.

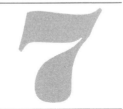

CHAPTER

Urinary Tract
Stone Disease

OBJECTIVES

After completing this chapter, you will be able to:

1. List the types of urinary calculi and describe their treatment

2. List the diagnostic procedures used in evaluation of urinary calculi

3. Identify the signs and symptoms of urinary calculi

4. Explain the process of crystallization and stone formation

5. Describe those persons at risk of forming urinary calculi.

A. Background

1. Incidence

Renal calculi, or stone disease, is a common problem. Each year, one person per thousand requires hospitalization for treatment of it. This number does not account for the many people who spontaneously pass stones with only minor symptoms. It has been estimated that 2 to 4 percent of all Americans will form renal calculi sometime. Stone disease is found in all parts of the world. In the United States, there is a higher incidence in the southeast coastal regions, and this area is sometimes referred to as the "stone belt."

Stone disease is seen mostly in adults between the ages of 20 and 40, with males having a higher incidence of the disease than females.

2. Stone formation

The formation of renal stones of any type involves crystallization. First, an organic matrix, which will comprise about 2.5 percent of the weight of the stone, is formed from mucoproteins. Crystalloids present in the urine bind onto the matrix to form a stone. Why urine supersaturates with a particular crystalloid is still under investigation. Although the exact cause of calculus formation is not clear, there are factors that seem to predispose a person to stone formation. These factors include high urine concentration caused either by dehydration or an increase in the crystalloid solutes that form stones, urinary stasis due to obstruction or immobilization, a family history of stone diseases, and certain metabolic disturbances that cause an increase of stone-forming solutes in the urine.

3. Types of calculi

a. Calcium stones. These are the most common type of renal stones. Approximately 90 percent of all renal calculi contain calcium of some sort, usually oxalate or phosphate (75 percent). Hypercalciuria, an increase of calcium solute in the urine, is seen in many people with calcium-forming stone disease. Hypercalciuria is caused by several factors:

- An increased reabsorption of calcium from bone results in hypercalciuria; conditions that cause calcium resorption are primary hyperparathyroidism, treatment of Cushing's disease (due to use of steroids), bone cancer, and immobilization
- Inability of kidney to excrete acid causes a metabolic acidosis (renal tubular acidosis), which results in a mobilization of calcium from bone
- Gastric bypass, excessive ingestion of vitamin D, and milk-alkali syndrome that occurs with some ulcer diets can cause increased absorption of calcium from the intestine
- Structural abnormalities, such as sponge kidney, may result in hypercalciuria.

Oxalate is a component of many of the calcium stones. It is insoluble in urine, and its role in stone formation is yet unclear. Dietary factors have been associated with calcium oxalate stone formation, in that people with a high-carbohydrate diet have an increased frequency of forming calcium stones.

There is also a rare condition known as primary hyperoxaluria, which causes high concentrations of oxalate in the urine and blood. It is due to an enzyme deficiency that may result in formation of oxalate.

b. Uric acid stones. These stones are formed as a result of urinary supersaturation with uric acid. Dehydration causes a low urine pH and an increase in uric acid formation, which provides the right condition for the formation of uric acid stones. Conditions that cause hyperuricuria are primary and secondary gout, ileostomy (due to decreased urine volume), leukemia, and lymphoma.

c. Cystine stones. Cystine stone formation is caused by supersaturation of the urine with cystine. Cystinuria results from an inherited inability of the renal tubes to absorb four amino acids, one of which is cystine, thereby causing large amounts of urinary cystine. Cystinuria, with consequent cystine stones, usually occurs in childhood, with the incidence decreasing in adulthood.

d. Miscellaneous. Xanthine stone formation is caused by a rare hereditary condition, a deficiency of the enzyme xanthine oxidase, that results in high blood and urine levels of xanthine.

Struvite (triple phosphate) stones are usually found in infected alkaline urine. Proteus, a urea-splitting organism, is most often the causative bacteria. Struvite stones are the major cause of staghorn calculus formation.

4. Ureteral calculi

Like renal calculi, ureteral stones occur more frequently in males. These stones are really renal calculi that are pushed along with peristalsis through the ureter. A stone that is too large to pass becomes lodged in the ureter. The narrow ureteropelvic junction is a common site for calculi to be found. Ureteral calculi may obstruct the ureter, causing hydronephrosis and infection. Symptoms include renal colic that radiates to the groin or perineum.

5. Bladder calculi

Stone formation also occurs in the bladder. Common causes of bladder calculi are urinary stasis and conditions that cause it, such as prostatic hypertrophy, bladder diverticuli, cystoceles, and neurogenic bladders. These calculi cause infections that persist so long as the stones are not removed. Pain and hematuria can be symptomatic of bladder calculi.

B. Assessment

Renal stones may form in the calyx of the kidney and remain asymptomatic or with only occasional hematuria. Stones in the renal pelvis frequently cause obstructions that lead to pain. Stones larger than 1 cm usually do not pass through the ureter.

1. Symptoms

a. Pain. Flank pain, which can be excruciating, is the hallmark symptom of any type of stone. The pain is commonly referred to as renal colic. Its onset can be sudden and is usually caused by dilation and/or obstruction of the ureter.

Pain from renal calculi is usually confined to the flank area, but may radiate to the abdomen, whereas ureteral calculi frequently cause pain that radiates to the groin.

b. Other symptoms. Hematuria may be present, due to tissue trauma caused by movement of the calculus. Infection caused by obstruction is also common in stone disease. Other symptoms include those associated with cystitis, such as urinary frequency, urgency, and dysuria.

2. Diagnostic studies

a. Clinical laboratory. Urine samples are analyzed for infection, hematuria, and pH. A 24-hour urine collection is done to detect any abnormal amounts of common stone-forming substances. It's important to strain the patient's urine during this time to detect any stones or particles of stone that might pass. Serum levels of calcium, uric acid, phosphorus, and other stone-forming substances are determined.

b. Radiology. Radiographic studies confirm the diagnosis and position of the stone. A kidney-ureter-bladder X-ray can detect 90 percent of urinary stones. Most stones are radiopaque because of their calcium content. An intravenous pyelogram is also usually performed to provide information on functioning of the kidney.

C. Treatment of urinary calculi

Usual management has been medical or surgical.

1. Medical management

Once calculi are diagnosed, they are followed by routine X-rays to evaluate for any increase. Any aggravated symptom is also important when treating calculi conservatively, because it may indicate that the stone is moving or getting larger and causing trauma.

Medical management usually consists of the following:

1. Encouragement of high fluid intake.

2. Dietary restriction of stone-forming substances:
- Calcium stones: Encourage an acid-ash diet, which acid-

ifies the urine and increases the solubility of calcium phosphate, and a low-calcium diet, restricting milk and dairy products
- Uric acid stones: Restrict purine (liver, kidney, seafoods, spinach)
- Cystine stones: Eliminate animal protein; encourage a high-vegetable diet.

3. Medications – some medications used in the treatment of stone diseases are:
- Calcium stones: Thiazides reduce the amount of calcium excreted in the urine; allopurinol (Lopurin, Zyloprim) decreases hyperuricosuria
- Uric acid stones: Urinary alkalizers such as sodium bicarbonate
- Cystine stones: Anticystinuric medications such as dpenicillamine.

4. Stone dissolution. Dissolution of renal calculi is accomplished by placement of a nephrostomy tube and administering one of the various solutions appropriate for the stone type. Renacidin is a commonly used solution.

This treatment may be used alone or in conjunction with manipulation. Because this method is slow and must be done over a long period, it is not popular. It is essential to control intrarenal pressure when irrigating directly into the kidney. An outflow system, or safety valve, should be in position on a pole 20 cm above the kidney during infusion.

2. Surgical management

Indications for surgical removal of a stone are infection, obstruction, a stone larger than 1 cm in diameter, persistent renal colic, and renal damage caused by the calculus. There are several techniques used in the removal of a calculus:

a. Percutaneous manipulation. A guide wire is manipulated through a percutaneous nephrostomy tube under fluoroscopy to dislodge the stone. If the stone is smaller than 1 cm it can be retrieved with forceps. Sometimes the kidney is flushed with saline solution to facilitate movement of the stone.

b. Percutaneous nephrostolithotomy. Percutaneous nephrostolithotomy is a relatively new and increasingly popular technique for removing stones from the upper urinary tract. It uses ultrasonic shock waves to fragment stones that are too large to be removed. The procedure is performed over a two-day period. First, a percutaneous nephrostomy tube is placed in the renal collecting system. With the patient in a prone position on the fluoroscopy table, a needle is inserted through the skin and directly into the kidney. Contrast medium is used to visualize the kidney and stone. A guide wire is then passed, and the needle removed. Progressively larger dilators are passed to form a tract, and a nephrostomy tube is inserted. The next day, under either local or general anesthesia, the tract is further dilated, and the stone is fragmented by ultrasonic energy.

X-rays are normally taken after the procedure to check for any fragments of stone not removed during the procedure. The nephrostomy tube is left in place for a day or two and then removed. The advantages of this procedure are that it has a decreased morbidity rate and requires less time for recovery. As a result, there is a shorter hospital stay and lower cost.

c. Cystoscopy. A bladder calculi can be removed with a basket that can expand to trap it. A stone can also be removed transurethrally by litholapaxy. The stone is crushed with a lithotrite and then removed with forceps or by basket extraction.

Ureteral calculi that do not pass spontaneously can be removed by endoscopic procedures if they are in the lower two-thirds of the ureter. Stones lodged higher in the ureter or too large to be removed by endoscopy may require ureterolithotomy, an open surgical procedure.

d. Ureterolithotomy. The location of the stone determines the incision site, but usually a flank incision is used in the procedure. Postoperative management includes the same nursing procedures employed for postoperative nephrectomy patients. A Penrose drain is usually left in place to allow drainage of urine that may leak from the incision in the ureter. Pouching the drain precludes frequent dressing changes and provides for more accurate assessment of the amount of drainage.

e. Other procedures. Two other open surgical procedures to remove renal calculi are the pyelolithotomy and nephrolithotomy. A pyelolithotomy is the removal of a stone from the renal parenchyma.

Partial nephrectomy is sometimes indicated if the kidney is damaged or if the stone is too large to be removed by the other methods. Staghorn calculi are generally the cause of such conditions.

3. Extracorporeal shock wave lithotripsy

This noninvasive treatment, developed in Germany and now being used in the United States, is the newest method of kidney stone destruction. The stones are disintegrated by shock waves produced outside the body by a high-voltage condensor spark discharge. The procedure is done with the patient immersed in a water bath, which allows the shock waves to enter the body. The crushed stones are passed with urine when the patient voids.

QUIZ

1. Formation of renal stones involves a process of
_____ on an organic matrix.

2. Stone disease occurs mostly in adults between the
ages of _____ and _____.

3. _____, _____,
_____,
and _____ are some predisposing
factors for the formation of urinary calculi.

4. _____ -containing stones are the most common types of calculi.

5. Stones larger than_____ usually do not pass through the ureter.

6. _____ is the major symptom of urinary calculi.

7. Medical management of stone disease consists of _____, _____, _____, and _____.

8. _____ is a new technique that is used to remove stones in the upper urinary tract by ultrasonic dissolution.

ANSWERS
1. Crystallization.
2. 20, 40.
3. High urine concentration, urinary stasis, family history of stone disease, metabolic disturbances.
4. Calcium.
5. 1 cm.
6. Flank pain.
7. High fluid intake, diet restriction, medication, stone dissolution.
8. Percutaneous nephrostolithotomy.

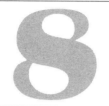

Disorders of the Male Reproductive System

OBJECTIVES

After completing this chapter, you will be able to:

1. *List the infectious, benign, and neoplastic disorders of the prostate*

2. *Understand how the various disorders of the prostate are diagnosed and treated*

3. *Describe the stages and grades of prostatic and testicular cancer and give the rationale for the different modes of treatment*

4. *Identify the disorders associated with the testicle and the treatment of these disorders*

5. *Identify the disorders of the penis and scrotum and treatment of these disorders.*

A. Disorders of the prostate

1. Benign prostatic hypertrophy (BPH)

BPH is the most common disorder of the prostate in men older than 45 years. With hyperplasia, or increased cell formation, in the prostatic tissue, the gland becomes larger. Since the prostate surrounds the urethra, any enlargement may interfere with urethral patency and urinary flow.

The etiology of BPH is unknown. Among the many proposed causes of prostatic hyperplasia are chronic inflammation and neoplastic, endocrinologic, arteriosclerotic, metabolic, and nutritional factors. The most common theory is that endocrine disturbances in the older male are the cause.

a. Signs and symptoms. With prostate gland compression of the posterior urethra, the patient experiences decreased urinary stream, nocturia, and urgency. When its outlet is obstructed, the bladder becomes continuously distended with urine. The distention eventually impairs the contractile ability of the bladder muscles and causes bladder decompensation, an inability of the bladder to further compensate for increased pressure. A reflux of urine into the ureters may occur, causing hydronephrosis and impaired renal function.

Some men have a silent prostatism with no early symptoms before they present with acute urinary retention or symptoms of renal impairment from decompensation.

b. Diagnosis. Palpation of the prostate in a rectal examination should show it to be firm and smooth. Since only the posterior lobe can be palpated, it may or may not indicate that the patient has an enlarged prostate.

A post-voiding residual can be performed to evaluate the bladder's ability to empty; any volume larger than 50 to 100 ml is abnormal. Urodynamic studies are done to evaluate the capacity, flow rates, and pressure gradients of the bladder.

Other procedures include blood studies (BUN and creatinine) and intravenous pyelogram. Urine cultures should be obtained to detect any infections. A cystoscopy may be performed on an outpatient basis.

c. Treatment. At this time, the only treatment available for BPH is surgical removal of the prostate. This is done when the patient has begun to develop bladder decompensation. Urinary retention, hydronephrosis, impaired renal function, and persistent urinary tract infections due to residual urine are indications for a prostatectomy.

The prostate can be removed in several different procedures. The most frequently used method is transurethral resection of the prostate (TURP). If the gland is too large to remove by this method, then an open approach has to be taken.

Open surgical methods include:

- suprapubic prostatectomy, in which a lower abdominal incision is made and the gland is removed or enucleated through the bladder neck;

- retropubic prostatectomy, which also requires a lower abdominal incision, but the gland is removed through the prostatic capsule, and no incision is made to the bladder; and

- a perineal prostatectomy, performed through an incision between the anus and scrotum. The gland is removed through the posterior part of the prostatic capsule. This is the least popular method of prostate gland removal because of the high rate of impotence after the procedure.

d. Assessment. Immediately postop, monitor the patient's vital signs frequently and watch the amount, quality, and character of drainage from the bladder. Initially expect bloody urine, which eventually clears. The catheter may need to be irrigated with physiologic saline solution to keep patent. Following removal of the suprapubic tube, assess the amount of drainage from that site, and after the bladder catheter is removed, keep track of the time, amount, and character of each urine specimen. At this time, it is important to prevent retention.

2. Prostatitis

Infectious processes of the prostate can be categorized as acute and chronic bacterial prostatitis, prostatitis caused by organisms other than bacteria, and prostatodynia.

a. Acute prostatitis. Prostatitis is a bacterial infection of the prostate gland. In acute prostatitis, the infection is located in the prostatic ducts and gland and is accompanied by purulent material. The causative organisms may be from the urethra, a urinary tract infection (ascending or descending), or from instrumentation used in some procedure on the urinary tract.

Symptoms of acute prostatitis include fever, chills, malaise, urinary frequency, sometimes urinary retention, low back pain, and perineal pain. On rectal exam, the prostate will feel enlarged and very tender.

Sitz baths and appropriate antibiotic therapy are used to treat acute prostatitis. The patient may require hospitalization to receive IV antibiotics. Massage of the prostate gland and catheterization should be avoided with these patients.

b. Chronic prostatitis. Chronic prostatitis is more common in men older than age 60. Symptoms are less severe than in the acute form, and usually a fever is not present. Many patients experience low back pain and a feeling of fullness in the perineum. These symptoms are believed to be caused by a stasis of the prostatic and seminal vesicle secretions. Prostatic secretion cultures are positive for the offending organism. In a rectal exam, the gland may feel boggy and indurated.

Sitz baths are helpful with chronic prostatitis. Unlike with acute prostatitis, prostatic massage may be helpful with this condition. Long-term antibiotic therapy is necessary. Successful treatment is extremely difficult to accomplish.

c. Nonbacterial prostatitis. Patients with prostatitis caused by organisms other than bacteria present much like those with prostatitis. Usually, they are not treated with antibiotics.

d. Prostatodynia prostatitis. In this condition, the patient experiences symptoms of prostatitis, but no inflammation is present. On rectal exam, the gland feels normal. The origin of prostatodynia is thought to be a neuromuscular dysfunction that causes spasm of the muscles around the prostate. Antispasmodics may be used as treatment.

B. Cancer of the prostate

Prostatic cancer is the most common cancer in men older than age 70, although the disease is seen in men as young as 50. It is the second most common cancer in males and is responsible for 10 percent of all cancer deaths in males.

Although the causes of prostatic cancer are not known, there are some factors that may contribute to the development of the disease. One theory suggests that androgens such as testosterone may contribute to prostatic hyperplasia, which is thought to be precancerous.

Sexual activity may also be a factor, in that males who have had many sexual partners, began sexual activity at an early age, or have had increased the frequency of intercourse may be predisposed to prostatic cancer.

Industrial workers exposed to cadmium are also at risk.

1. Signs and symptoms

Symptoms of prostatic cancer usually do not appear until the cancerous gland grows large enough to cause urinary obstruction. Symptoms of local metastases, such as low back pain from bone involvement, may appear first. The way to detect a cancerous prostatic lesion early is by rectal examination, which should be done yearly on men after age 45.

2. Diagnosis

a. Rectal examination. On rectal exam, a cancerous prostate feels hard and indurated. A needle biopsy, which is very accurate and often used, is then performed, either by the transrectal or transperineal approach. A transurethral biopsy of the gland may also be performed.

b. Serum acid phosphotase levels. These studies help determine the extent of metastasis, if any. Acid phosphotase is an enzyme secreted by the prostate. It becomes elevated in serum when the cancerous gland is unable to rid the enzyme through its ductal system. Acid phosphotase levels are usually normal when the tumor is confined to the prostate. Intravenous pyelogram is done to scan for obstructions or delayed filling.

c. Bone studies. Bone studies also help determine metastasis. A skeletal survey and scan are usually done, and sometimes a bone marrow biopsy is performed. Staging the prostatic cancer is also accomplished by lymphangiography. A staging lymphadenectomy may be done as a guide for therapy.

3. Staging and grading

The grading of a tumor establishes the activity of cancer, and staging defines the extent to which the disease has spread in the body. The stage and grade of the tumor help determine what treatment to use. There are several schemes used to stage prostatic cancer. One method is as follows:

- Stage A: Cancer is microscopic and confined inside the prostatic capsule
- Stage B: Cancer is a nodule, localized within the prostate gland
- Stage C: Cancer is found outside the prostate gland but localized within the pelvis
- Stage D: There are distant metastases outside the pelvic cavity, e.g., lymphatic involvement.

There are also different methods of grading, with three to five categories. One such method is as follows:

- Grade I: Well differentiated
- Grade II: Intermediate or moderately differentiated
- Grade III: Poorly differentiated.

4. Treatment

There are generally three modes of treatment for prostatic cancer: surgery, radiation, and drug therapy with hormones. Choice of treatment may vary from institution to institution, and most treatment protocols depend on the stage and grade of the tumor.

a. Radical prostatectomy. This surgery, which is done retropubically or perineally, is usually reserved for Stage A and Stage B tumors that are confined to the prostate. A transurethral prostatectomy is indicated in Stages C and D for palliative treatment if bladder outlet obstruction occurs.

b. Pelvic lymphadenectomy with ^{125}I implantation. This therapy is employed for localized (Stage B) tumor.

Radioactive implants cause less bowel and bladder irritation than does external radiation, and less normal tissue is damaged by it. In Stage C, it is followed by external radiation. One advantage of lymphadenectomy is that the disease can be staged and treated in one procedure.

c. Bilateral orchiectomy. This procedure is sometimes performed in conjunction with hormonal therapy to deprive the cancer cells of testosterone. It usually is done only in Stage D.

d. External radiation. This mode of treatment is used sometimes for Stage B tumors and Stage C tumors, following a pelvic lymphadenectomy. Although there are improved methods and machines that can concentrate the radiation more directly on the prostate, there are still complications of gastrointestinal and genitourinary irritation and sexual impotence associated with external radiation.

e. Endocrine therapy. It has been shown that prostatic cancer cells are androgen-dependent and die when testosterone is removed from the system. This is the rationale for reducing testosterone levels either by castration (orchiectomy) or through the use of estrogens or a combination of both. Diethylstilbestrol is the drug commonly used to suppress serum testosterone. Progesterone drugs such as megestrol (Megace, Pallace) and hydroxyprogesterone (Delalutin) are also used. Hormonal treatment is generally confined to Stage D cancer.

C. Disorders of the testicle

1. Infections of the spermatic cord

a. Epididymitis. The vas and epididymis can be infected by hematogenous spread of the pathogen or by its movement from a lower urinary tract or prostatic infection. Venereal diseases may also cause the infection. With epididymitis, the scrotum is usually swollen, erythematous, tender, and very painful.

Treatment includes the use of antibiotics, ice packs to the scrotum, scrotal elevation, and bed rest. Response to therapy is generally good, but occasionally this condition leads to the formation of an abscess.

b. Orchitis. Orchitis is an infection in the testicle. It can be caused by a bacterial organism secondary to epididymitis or during mumps in an adult. Symptoms are similar to those found in epididymitis. Corticosteroids are sometimes used to reduce the inflammation. Other interventions include scrotal elevation, ice packs, and bed rest.

2. Testicular torsion

Torsion of the testicle is considered a urologic emergency, and prompt treatment is essential if the testicle is to be salvaged. Torsion is seen up to young adulthood and most often before puberty.

With testicular torsion, the cord becomes twisted and deprives the testicle of venous drainage and arterial supply, causing swelling, edema, and eventually necrosis. Symptoms include severe pain and tenderness in the scrotal area, usually sudden in onset. Treatment is immediate surgery to untwist the cord and restore blood supply to the testis. If during surgery a testis is found to be necrotic, it is removed at that time. The testicle on the unaffected side may be fixed in place (orchiopexy) to prevent torsion of it.

3. Trauma

Blunt trauma to the scrotal area does not often result in injury to the testes because of their mobility. Damage may occur in the form of intrascrotal hematoma or testicular hematoma. In some cases, scrotal exploration may be necessary to drain the hematoma and relieve pressure from the testicle. For simple contusions, treatment consists of ice packs, scrotal elevation, and bed rest until symptoms subside.

D. Testicular cancer

Testicular cancer is the most serious and most common cancer seen in young males between the ages of 25 and 40 years. It is estimated that two cases per 100,000 are diagnosed yearly (approximately 2,500 new cases). Blacks and Asians have a very low incidence of testicular cancer.

Based on origin, the tumors can be classified in two types, germ cell and nongerm cell carcinoma, with the germinal tumors comprising 95 percent of the cases.

The germinal cell tumors are further categorized into:
- seminomas — 40-45 percent, least malignant;
- embryonic carcinomas — 20 percent, second most common;
- teratomas — 20 percent, third most common; and
- choriocarcinomas — 2-5 percent, least common, most malignant.

Nongerminal tumors usually originate from Leydig's and Sertoli's cells.

1. Signs and symptoms

Seventy percent of men with testicular cancer report a pain-less swelling of the testicle. Only approximately 10 percent experience pain in the testicle. Other symptoms may include gynecomastia and back pain from lymph node involvement.

2. Diagnosis and staging

Physical examination of the testis shows a hard mass that will not transilluminate in the dark, since it is not fluid-filled. Tumor diagnosis is made by an exploration and radical orchiectomy by inguinal approach. Scrotal incisions must be avoided with suspected testicular cancer to prevent any further lymphatic contamination with cancer cells. The scrotum and testes drain into different lymphatics.

Many methods are utilized in the staging of testicular cancer: chest X-rays and lung tomograms, routine serum studies, intravenous pyelogram, abdominal CAT scan, lymphangiogram, inferior venacavogram (if there is suspicion of vena cava involvement), biochemical serum markers (alpha-fetoprotein and the beta subunit of human chorionic gonadotropin) that frequently elevate with malignant cancer and return to normal if there is a remission in the disease. These serum markers serve as important monitors of the disease after treatment.

Testicular tumors can be staged as follows:
- Stage I: Tumor is not found beyond the testis

- Stage II: Tumor involves testis and has spread to retro-peritoneal lymph nodes
- Stage III: There are metastases beyond retroperitoneal lymph nodes.

3. Treatment

Depending on the type and stage of the disease, testicular tumors are treated with surgery, X-ray, and chemotherapy. All primary tumors, regardless of the type, are removed by radical orchiectomy.

a. Pure seminomas. If detected early enough, these are usually successfully treated with orchiectomy, followed by radiation to surrounding lymph nodes. Stage II seminomas are treated with higher doses of radiation after orchiectomy. Stage III seminomas are sometimes treated with chemotherapy instead of radiation.

b. Embryonic carcinomas, choriocarcinomas, and tera-tocarcinomas. These are generally treated by radical orchiectomy and retroperitoneal lymphadenectomy, followed by chemotherapy if the tumor could not be removed completely. These tumors have a low rate of response to radiation therapy.

With improvements in chemotherapeutic agents, the survival rate for testicular cancer has reached 80 to 90 percent. The combined use of cisplatin (Platinol), vinblastine (Velban), and bleomycin (Blenoxane), has been particularly successful. Actinomycin D and cyclophosphamide (Cytoxan) are also used in some regimens. Nursing care during chemotherapy includes assessment for response to treatment and for adverse effects of the cytotoxic drugs.

In order to detect testicular cancer early, all men should be taught self-examination of the testicles. Resources such as material distributed by the American Cancer Society are helpful in teaching men this procedure.

E. Disorders of the penis

1. Priapism

Priapism is uncontrolled, prolonged erection of the penis, unrelated to sexual activity or arousal. The erection involves only the corpora cavernosa, with the corpus spongiosum remaining unengorged. Venous drainage becomes blocked, and the blood in the corpora stagnates. Resulting decreased oxygenation to the corpora eventually causes fibrosis and impotence.

There are various causes for priapism. Sickle cell disease, prolonged sexual activity, leukemia, and spinal cord injuries are considered predisposing factors. Treatment depends on the underlying cause, but usually involves one or more of the following: sedatives, anticoagulants, warm or cold enemas, spinal anesthesia, and needle aspiration of the corpora. If these conservative measures fail, then surgery is indicated to shunt and drain the penis.

2. Hydrocele

This common condition is a collection of serous fluid inside the tunica vaginalis or around the testis or both. The sac may extend up the spermatic cord, but this is rare. Hydroceles produce a soft painless mass that transilluminates when light is directed at the scrotum in a darkened room. The condition is thought to be caused by an overproduction of secretions from the tunica vaginalis. Diagnosis is made by transillumination, CAT scan, and/or needle aspiration, which usually produces a clear, yellowish fluid. Although needle aspiration can be used as a treatment, surgical excision is usually necessary.

3. Urethral strictures

A stricture or narrowing of the urethra with consequent obstruction or decreased flow of urine is due to scar tissue or fibrous replacement of normal mucosa. Trauma to the urethra or infection may be the underlying cause. Infection-induced strictures are commonly associated with gonococcal infection or urethritis. Trauma to the urethra may occur with crushing injury to the pelvis or during instrumentation procedures such as catheterization or cystoscopy. The bladder eventually experiences decompensation due to the constant pressure on its muscles to overcome the obstruction. Hydronephrosis and decreased renal function are sequelae of this process.

a. Diagnosis. The most common symptom of a stricture is a decrease in the urinary stream, followed by the signs of obstruction (hydronephrosis, decreased renal function, infection). A urethrography or cystoscopy may be performed to confirm the diagnosis.

b. Treatment. Urethral strictures may be treated by dilation with various filiforms and catheters.

Most patients require surgical intervention, and internal urethrotomy is the most commonly used procedure. It allows for direct visualization of the urethra, and the stricture is excised with little or no trauma to the healthy tissue. Large strictures require more complicated technique, done in two procedures and employing grafts.

QUIZ

1. A common benign disorder of the prostate in older men is _____.

2. Bladder decompensation occurs in _____
_____, when the bladder muscles loose their contractile ability.

3. On physical exam, a normal prostate should feel _____ and _____ whereas a cancerous prostate will feel _____ and
_____.

4. _____ is the surgical treatment of choice for prostatic cancer.

5. The rationale for endocrine therapy in prostatic cancer is that the prostatic cancer cells are thought to be _____ -dependent and die when deprived of _____.

6. Orchitis is sometimes a secondary complication of _____ in the adult.

7. _____ of the testis is a serious complication of testicular torsion.

8. Based on cell origin, testicular tumors can be classified into two types _____ and _____ _____ with _____ comprising 95 percent of cases.

9. _____ is a condition of the penis in which there is an uncontrolled, prolonged erection, unrelated to sexual activity.

10. The usual causes of urethral strictures are _____ and _____.

ANSWERS
  1. Benign prostatic hypertrophy.
  2. Bladder outlet obstruction.
  3. Firm, smooth, hard, indurated.
  4. Radical prostatectomy.
  5. Androgen, testosterone.
  6. Mumps.
  7. Necrosis.
  8. Germinal, nongerminal, germinal.
  9. Priapism.
10. Infection, trauma.

C H A P T E R

Male Sexual Dysfunction

OBJECTIVES

After completing this chapter, you will be able to:

1. *Describe the organic causes of impotence*

2. *Understand the medical and surgical interventions used to treat the impotent male*

3. *List the laboratory and surgical tests used in the evaluation of male infertility*

4. *Identify the treatments commonly used for male infertility.*

A. Introduction

Sexuality is a part of everyday life, and regardless of its expression, is an important component of health.

Nurses caring for male urology patients sometimes have a difficult and perhaps embarrassing task. These patients are frequently faced with the prospect of some change in their sexuality. They — older men, particularly — may be sensitive to verbalizing their sexual fears or problems with a female nurse. Dealing effectively with such patients requires an atmosphere of trust between nurse and patient. You must, so to say, earn the patient's permission to discuss this subject with him.

This chapter deals with the two most frequently encountered sexual dysfunctions among urology patients: impotence and infertility. But remember that sexual problems among urology patients are certainly not limited to these two disorders. Patients with carcinoma, hydroceles, and the other disorders described in Chapter 8 may also experience a change in sexuality, which must be considered in developing a plan of care for them.

B. Impotence

1. Etiology

Impotence is the inability to maintain or achieve an erection sufficient for sexual intercourse. Most men experience impotence at some time in their lives, but only once in a while. Patients who are impotent either often or always over a considerable period may seek medical help.

a. Current diagnostic approach. These men who seek help are frequently referred to a urologist, who attempts to find an organic cause for the condition. Many medical centers have impotence evaluation centers that use a multidisciplinary team approach, including the urologist, an endocrinologist and/or internist, and a psychologist or psychiatrist who specializes in sexual counseling.

In the not-too-distant past, physicians considered about 90 percent of all cases of impotence to be psychological in origin. Research into the problem of impotence has more recently revealed that this figure has been a gross over-exaggeration. Although many cases of impotence are psychological in origin, a great many disease conditions or surgical interventions as well as certain medications can lead to organic impotence.

2. Physiology of the normal erection

The corpora cavernosa of the penis are what produce an erection. Each of the corpora is surrounded first by a strong fibrous sheath and then by the ischiocavernosus muscles, finally by the tunica albuginea. Blood supply to the penis comes from the internal iliac artery, and nerve supply is from the somatic and parasympathetic fibers of cord roots S_2 to S_4. Neurogenic cerebral input may also affect ability to achieve erection. All of these anatomic factors must be intact for erection to take place.

a. Process of erection. Muscle fibers that lie longitudinally in the small arteries and veins of the penis play an important role in erection. When the penis is flaccid, these muscles maintain venous drainage. During erection, arterial muscles relax and venous muscles close to prevent venous flow, which engorges the blood vessels and produces erection. The ischiocavernosus muscles aid in keeping the penis rigid, but not in creating or maintaining an erection.

b. Organic causes of impotence. As can be seen in Table 9-1, inflammatory, endocrinologic, metabolic, neurologic, traumatic, vascular, neoplastic, and congenital disorders as well as the effects of certain medications can cause impotence. Therefore, a thorough medical, neurologic, and vascular evaluation is necessary to rule out such organic causes.

3. Evaluation

Physical examination is the first step in evaluating the patient with impotence. The physician looks for symptoms suggestive of an underlying disorder. Initially, vascular supply can be evaluated by palpating the dorsal penile artery pulse. Neurologic status can be partially ascertained by check-

TABLE 9-1
CAUSES OF ORGANIC IMPOTENCE

Inflammatory
Cystitis
Ileofemoral arteritis
Peripheral neuritis
Peyronie's disease
Prostatitis
Seminal vesiculitis
Urethral stricture
Urethritis

Endocrinologic
Acromegaly
Addison's disease
Cushing's syndrome
Diabetes mellitus
Fröhlich's syndrome
Hyperthyroidism
Hypogonadism
Hypothyroidism
Laurence-Moon-Biedl
   syndrome

Metabolic
Hepatic cirrhosis
Renal failure

Neurologic
Alzheimer's disease
Amyotrophic lateral sclerosis
Cord compression
Multiple sclerosis
Pernicious anemia
Spina bifida
Syringomyelia
Tabes dorsalis
Temporal lobe epilepsy

Traumatic
Abdominal perineal resection
Castration
Cystectomy
Head trauma
Lymphadenectomy
Pelvic fracture
Pelvic irradiation
Perineal biopsies
Postvascular surgery
Prostatectomy
Spinal cord trauma
Sympathectomy (dorsal,
   lumbar, pelvic)
Urethral rupture

Vascular
Iliac artery obstruction
Leriche's syndrome
Priapism
Senility

Neoplastic
Adrenal tumor
Hypothalamic tumor
Pituitary tumor
Spinal cord tumor
Squamous cell cancer of penis

Congenital
Epispadias
Hypospadias
Microphallus

Pharmacologic
Antihistamines
Antihypertensives
Barbiturates
Bromides
Cimetidine
Dilantin
Estrogen
Ethanol
MAO inhibitors
Morphine
Parasympatholytics
Sympatholytics
Tranquilizers

ing the anal and bulbocavernosus reflexes. The lower genito-urinary tract is examined for obvious abnormalities. Urinalysis looks for evidence of inflammation.

a. Laboratory studies. Laboratory studies commonly performed include complete blood count, blood chemistries, glucose levels, serum testosterone, and prolactin. Blood chemistries and glucose levels can detect various metabolic or endocrine disorders. Serum testosterone and prolactin levels also help to detect endocrine disorders. Routine genito-urinary studies – intravenous pyelogram and cystoscopy – rule out anatomic abnormalities.

b. Referrals. Patients with abnormal blood studies are referred to an appropriate specialist. For example, patients with high glucose levels should be evaluated for diabetes, and patients with high prolactin levels should be referred to an endocrinologist. Patients with low serum testosterone levels may receive supplemental injections of testosterone enanthate (Delatestryl). Usually follicle stimulating hormone and luteinizing hormone levels are also drawn on these patients.

c. Vascular studies. Vascular supply to the penis can be evaluated by a Doppler study of the penile arteries, comparing systolic pressure in them to brachial artery systolic pressure. Penile arteriography is sometimes used when severe vascular disease is present. However, surgical revascularization, or bypasses of atherosclerotic arteries of the penis, is rarely performed. This surgery is currently performed by only a few physicians in this country.

d. Nocturnal penile tumescence (NPT) testing. This is a valuable tool in differentiating between organic and psychogenic impotence. Normally, men have between three and five nonsexual erections during the REM period of sleep. With transducers attached to the base and tip of the penis, erectile and expansive properties of the penis during sleep are monitored. If normal nonsexual erections are found to occur, impotence is most likely not organic in origin, and a psychogenic cause should be suspected.

e. Psychological evaluation. If the results of these examinations are all normal, the physician may refer the patient for psychological evaluation. It is not uncommon for urologists to have impotence patients take the Minnesota Multiphasic Personality Inventory (MMPI) or a similar test prior to referral for counseling.

Patients are not usually told that their impotence is psychogenic unless all prior tests are normal. If there is any doubt about the origin of the impotence, further evaluation is indicated.

4. Treatment

If all studies performed on the patient during evaluation for impotence disclose nothing that can be corrected medically or show an organic cause for impotence that cannot be corrected, surgical intervention may be considered. In this case, too, NPT testing must reveal that nonsexual erections are not present, which means that psychological or sexual counseling is not indicated.

With the exception of the rarely done vascular surgery mentioned above, surgery for impotence involves implantation of one of several types of penile prostheses. Table 9-2 outlines the advantages and disadvantages of these prostheses.

a. Semirigid rod prosthesis. The Small-Carrion-, the Finney-, and Jonas-type prostheses are the most commonly used semirigid rod devices. These consist of two filled silicone rods that are implanted in the corpora cavernosa. A vertical suprapubic or a perineal incision is made to enable implantation. The spongy interior of the corpora is cleared away, and the prostheses are inserted bilaterally.

Postoperatively, the patient must usually have an indwelling Foley catheter for a short period. The incision is covered with a small dressing. Edema is ordinarily minimal. Hospital stay may be only for two days. Some centers perform this surgery on an outpatient basis. The result of this surgery is a penis that is always semierect. The patient can bend the penis upward for full erection and intromission.

TABLE 9-2

COMPARISON OF PENILE PROSTHESES

	Semirigid rod prosthesis	Inflatable prosthesis
Advantages	Shorter hospital stay Shorter recuperation No moving parts Less expensive	Simulates normal erections Flaccid penis when deflated No need to disguise
Disadvantages	Permanent semierect penis Difficult to disguise Possible erosion Possible infection	Longer hospital stay Longer recuperation period Possible mechanical failure requiring additional surgery Need to learn how to operate More expensive Possible infection Possible erosion

b. Inflatable penile prosthesis. This type of prosthesis was originally developed in 1972 and has been improved considerably since then. Thousands of these implants are now done annually, with complication rates decreasing.

This prosthesis consists of two hollow silicone cylinders, a reservoir filled with contrast solution, and an inflate-deflate pump. The cylinders are implanted into the corpora cavernosa, the reservoir under the rectus muscle in the abdomen, and the pump into the scrotum. All of these are connected by silicone tubing. The entire surgical procedure is performed through a suprapubic or scrotal incision.

Postoperatively, the patient will need an indwelling Foley catheter for several days. The incision is dressed, and edema is more marked than it is for surgery to implant a semirigid prothesis. Hospital stay is about five days. The patient needs to be taught to locate the pump in his scrotum and pull it gently downward in the scrotal sac once daily. He must also learn to depress the deflate valve on the pump at the same time, as gravity drainage of small amounts of fluid from the reservoir into the cylinders may occur during the four-to-six week postoperative period. Pulling down on the pump helps to position it in a place in the scrotum where the patient has easy access to it, before scar tissue forms around the pump. Depressing the deflate valve is necessary to promote proper fluid mechanics of the system and formation of scar tissue around a full reservoir, rather than one that is partially deflated.

c. Postoperative assessment. After either of these surgeries, assess your patient for pain, which is quite severe initially, requiring narcotic analgesia. Mild pain is common for several weeks after the initial postoperative period. Edema gradually subsides.

Patients with semirigid protheses can have intercourse sooner than those with inflatable prostheses. After implantation of the inflatable prosthesis, inflation is not usually attempted – except by the physician – until four to six weeks after the surgery. The first inflation by the patient is done in the physician's office so the doctor or nurse can instruct him on how to inflate and deflate the device.

5. Nursing implications

a. The patient's partner. If at all possible, the patient's sexual partner should be included in the patient's impotence evaluation. This is particularly important if the impotence is judged to be psychological in origin, as joint counseling can be very successful. If organic impotence is diagnosed and surgery is considered, the partner should be included in the decision to have surgery and in the choice of prosthesis. To date, studies done on postoperative partner satisfaction indicate success.

b. Preoperative planning. Planning care for the patient admitted for impotence surgery must begin preoperatively. Thorough explanations of preoperative preparations for surgery and postoperative expectations are needed and should include the patient's partner if possible.

c. Attitude toward patient. Always remember that restoration of sexuality represents a return to normal functioning for this patient. Many of these patients are well past middle age, and should not be regarded as "dirty old men." Rather, they are neurologically impaired, diabetic, or post-trauma patients who have elected to undergo surgery so that they may continue a pleasurable part of their lives.

C. Male infertility

The evaluation for infertility in the male is indicated when a couple have been unsuccessful in accomplishing pregnancy after 12 to 18 months of unprotected intercourse. It has been estimated that 49 percent of fertility disorders are secondary to problems in the male. A fertility evaluation for the male is simpler and less invasive than for the female. Therefore, it may be the male who undergoes evaluation initially.

1. Etiology

The urologist who evaluates the male for infertility or subfertility looks for factors that may affect spermatogenesis or transport of mature sperm through the appropriate pathways.

a. Normal physiology. In normal sperm production and transport, spermatozoa are produced in the testes; from the testes, sperm pass through the epididymis, vas deferens, and seminal vesicles. At ejaculation, sperm and secretions – the semen – are ejected out the urethra. Obviously, all of these pathways must be patent in order for the male to be fertile.

b. Conditions affecting fertility. Causes of infertility or subfertility are related to factors affecting the transport of sperm from testes to urethra or to factors affecting potency and ejaculation. Table 9-3 lists some of the many conditions that can affect fertility in the male.

2. Evaluation

a. Physical examination. Initially, the patient undergoes physical examination, with particular attention paid to the genital organs. The examiner looks for signs of systemic disease or endocrine disorders. When examining the genitalia,

TABLE 9-3

FACTORS AFFECTING FERTILITY IN THE MALE

Disorders of semen
Cryptorchidism
Varicocele
Sexual disorders
Anatomic disorders
Hypospadias
Testicular atrophy
Urethral strictures
Infection
Cystitis
Prostatitis
Seminal vesiculitis
Tuberculosis
Venereal disease
Endocrine disorders
Adrenal dysfunction
Diabetes
Hypogonadotropism
Hypothalamic dysfunction
Pituitary dysfunction
Thyroid dysfunction
Chromosomal abnormalities
Down's syndrome
Klinefelter's syndrome
Reifenstein's syndrome

Diseases
Allergies
Cancer
Liver dysfunction
Renal disease
Viral illnesses

Stress
Nutritional deficiencies
Age
Radiation
Heat
Medications
Substance abuse
Smoking

the penis and scrotum are evaluated for their size and appearance. The testicles and vas deferens are palpated bilaterally. The scrotum is carefully examined for the presence of a varicocele — an enlargement of the veins of the spermatic cord — appearing as a fullness on one side of the scrotum, usually the left, and feeling like a bundle of worms. Varicoceles can lead to subfertility for a variety of reasons, resulting in premature sloughing of spermatozoa in 90 percent of patients.

b. History. The sexual history of the couple is taken, sometimes with the help of a questionnaire. Medical history includes any previous genitourinary surgery or disorders, recent febrile illnesses and concomitant illnesses, any medications taken regularly, alcohol and drug use, and a family history. A history of cryptorchidism is especially important, as testes undescended by age 5 are infertile.

3. Semen analysis

Semen analysis is an essential part of the infertility evaluation. The semen specimen is collected after a period of sexual abstinence that corresponds to the frequency of intercourse by the couple. Collection is usually by masturbation.

a. Volume and viscosity. The semen is first evaluated for volume and viscosity. Semen ordinarily becomes coagulated after ejaculation, but liquefies after 20 minutes. Normal semen volume is 2 to 5 ml after three to five days of abstinence. Semen pH is also determined. Semen is alkaline, with a pH of 7.4 to 7.6.

b. Density. Microscopic examination of the semen estimates sperm density. Abnormal organisms (pyospermia) or imma- ture spermatozoa may be detected. The number of sperm cells is determined. Normally, there are 40 to 60 million sperm per cc. Oligospermia refers to decreased sperm cell count, azoospermia to the absence of sperm. Polyzoospermia may be present, with greater than 250 million sperm per cc.

c. Motility. Sperm motility is very important in estimating potential for fertility; 60 percent of the sperm should demon- strate activity or motility two hours after ejaculation. Ade- quate sperm motility depends on normal spermatogenesis and function of the epididymis, transportability through the vas deferens, and secretions of the seminal vesicles and prostate that increase motility and viability of the sperm. Viability of the sperm refers to the percentage of mature, normal sperm in the sperm cell count. Normally, 60 percent of the sperm are viable.

   If abnormalities are discovered in the semen analysis, fur- ther evaluations are done to attempt to pinpoint the disorder. Additional tests include:

   • Seminal fructose to evaluate the function and patency of the seminal vesicles and vas deferens (fructose is a product of the seminal vesicles)

- Seminal plasma zinc levels to evaluate prostatic secretions and
- Split ejaculate to evaluate which half of the ejaculate contains the greater sperm cell count (normally the greatest number of viable sperm are in the first one-third of the ejaculate).

4. Other diagnostic measures

a. Scrotal exploration and testicular biopsy. These are relatively simple minor surgical procedures that can reveal much about duct patency and testicular function. If results from a testicular biopsy are normal, ductal obstruction is usually suspected as the cause of infertility. If the biopsy shows abnormal results, various conditions that may prevent maturation or production of sperm or cause premature sloughing of sperm can be detected. Complications of testicular biopsy include infection, hematoma, and temporary decrease of spermatogenesis.

b. Endocrine evaluation. Serum testosterone, luteinizing hormone, and follicle stimulating hormone levels may aid in diagnosing an endocrine disorder that causes infertility. If these levels are abnormal, the patient may be referred to an endocrinologist.

Finally, chromosomal analysis may also be recommended.

5. Treatment

Correction of male infertility depends on the causative disorder. If permanent testicular damage is present and azoospermia is confirmed, little or nothing can be done.

a. Varicocelectomy. In case of varicocele, varicocelectomy may restore fertility. This surgical procedure involves division and ligation of the internal spermatic veins. Overnight hospitalization is usually required, and complications are minor, possibly including later development of a hydrocele.

b. Vasectomy reversal. Patients who have previously had a vasectomy and desire to become fertile again may undergo a vasovasostomy or vasoepididymostomy, a microscopic surgical procedure with success rates of up to 80 percent.

c. Life-style influences. Patients may be counseled regarding their sexual practices, use of medications and alcohol, and nutrition. The scrotum should not be exposed to increased heat, as normal testicular function requires the cooler-than-body-temperature environment of the scrotum. Hot baths, saunas, and tight clothing should be avoided.

d. Medications. Infectious processes of the lower genitourinary tract should be treated with appropriate antibiotics. Decreased volume may improve with injections of human chorionic gonadotropin (HCG). Steroids or HCG may improve motility. Hormonal and endocrine disorders may be treated according to the absent or decreased hormone or by treating the underlying condition.

QUIZ

1. Normal erection takes place primarily in the
_____ of the penis.

2. A test that helps to differentiate between organic and psychological impotence is _____
_____.

3. The penile prosthesis that creates a permanent semi-erect state is called the _____
prosthesis.

4. Inflatable penile prostheses are inflated via a pump located in the _____ .

5. Sperm are normally produced in the _____.

6. Secretions from the _____ and the _____ form part of the ejaculate, or semen.

7. Testes undescended by age _____ will be unable to produce sperm.

8. Enlargement of the veins of the spermatic cord is called _____.

9. Normal sperm cell count is from _____ to _____ million per cc.

10. Sperm motility refers to _____ of sperm cells several hours after ejaculation.

ANSWERS

1. Corpora cavernosa.
2. Nocturnal penile tumescence.
3. Semirigid rod.
4. Scrotum.
5. Testes.
6. Seminal vesicles, prostate.
7. 5.
8. Varicocele.
9. 40, 60.
10. Activity.

GLOSSARY

Anuria – absence of urine output

Bacteriuria – presence of bacteria in urine

BUN (blood urea nitrogen) – blood test that determines kidney function; an elevated BUN indicates abnormal renal function

Calculi – abnormal concentration of mineral salts, resulting in stone formation

Catheter – hollow plastic or rubber tube used to drain urine

Chordee – downward bowing of the penis

Coude catheter – catheter with an elbow curve at the tip

Creatinine – blood test that determines kidney function; an increased creatinine indicates damage to the nephrons

Crede's method – pressing inward on the lower abdomen in order to express urine

Cryptorchidism – undescended testicle

Cystectomy – surgical removal of the bladder

Cystinuria – congenital disorder resulting in excess urinary excretion of cystine and cystine calculi

Cystitis – infection of the bladder

Cystocele – prolapse of the bladder into the anterior vagina

Cystolithotomy – removal of calculi from the bladder

Cystometrography – test of bladder pressure and capacity

Cystoscopy – direct visualization of the inside of the bladder

Cystostomy – formation of an opening into the bladder

Detrusor – bladder muscle that contracts during voiding

Dysuria – burning pain on urination

Enuresis – incontinence at night without awakening (bedwetting)

Epididymitis – inflammation of the epididymis

Epispadias – congenital defect in which the meatus is located on the dorsal side of the penis

Glomerulonephritis – inflammation of the capillary loops in the glomeruli of the kidney

Hematospermia – presence of blood in the semen

Hematuria – presence of blood in the urine

Hydrocele – collection of fluid in a sac surrounding a testicle

Hydronephrosis – enlargement of the renal pelvis and calyces

Hypercalciuria – increased calcium in the urine

Hypernephroma – carcinoma of the kidney; renal cell carcinoma

Hyperuricuria – excess uric acid in the urine

Impotence – inability to achieve or maintain an erection

Incontinence – involuntary loss of urine

Intravenous pyelogram (or urogram) – radiologic study of the kidneys and ureters

Lithotrite – instrument used for crushing calculi

Nephrectomy – surgical removal of a kidney

Nephrolithotomy – surgical removal of stones located in the kidney

Nephrostomy – insertion of a catheter into the renal pelvis

Nephroureterectomy – surgical removal of the kidney and its ureter

Nocturia – urinary frequency at night

Nonseminoma – a classification of germ-cell testicular tumors; nonseminoma tumors are embryonic carcinomas, teratomas and choriocarcinomas

Orchiectomy – removal of a testis

Orchiopexy – surgical correction of an undescended testicle, placing the testicle in a normal scrotal position

Orchitis – inflammation of a testis

Paraphimosis – contraction of the foreskin so that it cannot be replaced over the glans penis

Phimosis – tightness of the foreskin so that it cannot be drawn back over the glans penis

Priapism – prolonged, usually painful erection not associated with sexual desire

Prostatectomy – surgical removal of all or part of the prostate gland

Prostatism – urethral obstruction secondary to prostatic enlargement

Prostatodynia – pain in the prostate gland

Proteinuria – presence of protein, usually albumin, in the urine

Pyelitis – inflammation of the pelvis of the kidney

Pyelolithotomy – removal of renal calculi from the pelvis of the kidney

Pyelonephritis – inflammation of the kidney and its pelvis

Pyuria – pus in the urine

Resectoscope – an instrument used for transurethral prostatic resection

Retrograde ejaculation – discharge of seminal fluid into the bladder rather than through the urethra; a condition usually present after prostatectomy

Retrograde pyelogram – injection of contrast material into the renal pelvis through ureteral catheters

Retrograde urethrogram – injection of contrast material into the urethra

Retropubic prostatectomy – enucleation of the prostate gland, using a suprapubic incision into the anterior surgical capsule of the prostate

Seminoma – a germ-cell tumor of the testis

Spermatocele – a cystic tumor of the epididymis, containing seminal fluid

Staghorn – a type of renal calculus that is branched into the renal pelvis and calyces

Strangury – difficult, painful urination produced by spasmodic muscular contraction of the urethra and the bladder

Stricture (urethral) – a partial or complete narrowing of the urethra

Suprapubic prostatectomy – enucleation of the prostate gland, using a suprapubic incision into the bladder

Torsion – a twisting of the testis that interferes with blood supply

TURP (transurethral resection of the prostate) – surgical removal of the enlarged portion of the prostate

Ureteroileostomy – urinary diversion procedure consisting of implantation of the ureters into a segment of ileum

Ureterolithotomy – removal of a calculus by incision into the ureter

Ureteroneocystostomy – reimplantation of the ureter into the bladder

Urethritis – inflammation of the urethra

Urethroplasty – plastic surgery repair to the urethra

Urethrotome – an instrument used for incision of a urethral stricture

ADDITIONAL TEST QUESTIONS

1. The three major areas of the kidney are the

_____, _____, and _____.

2. The renal pyramids lie within the _____
of the kidney.

3. The functional unit of the kidney is the _____.

4. The clump of capillaries that makes up a part of the
nephron is called the _____.

5. Urine travels down the ureter by _____.

6. The comma-shaped structure on the posterior
lateral surface of the testis is called the _____.

7. Sperm formed in the testes pass into the _____,
through the _____
to the seminal vesicles, and then into the _____
urethra.

8. A distended bladder sounds _____ to
percussion, whereas an empty bladder sounds

_____.

9. Ectopic ureters that empty into the vagina cause

_____.

10. Ectopic kidneys are usually located in the _____.

11. A radical nephrectomy includes excision of the
_____ and _____.

12. In hypospadias, the meatal opening of the urethra is
on the _____ side of the penile shaft.

13. _____ is an infectious condition of the kidney involving the renal parenchyma and collecting systems.

14. _____ is a kidney abscess that is confined in the renal cortex.

15. Four kinds of urinary incontinence are _____, _____, _____, and _____.

16. Blood in the semen is called _____.

17. _____ is the most frequently seen symptom of bladder cancer.

18. Herniation of the bladder mucosa through the bladder wall is called a _____.

19. A common postoperative complication of transurethral resection of the prostate is _____ _____.

20. Bogginess or enlargement of the prostate can indicate _____.

21. The _____ area of the spinal cord is the reflex neurogenic center for voiding.

22. The bladder muscle that controls voiding is the _____.

23. Direct visualization of the interior of the bladder is done by _____.

24. Cystitis in women is associated with _____, _____, and _____.

25. Prolapse of the bladder into the anterior vagina is a _____.

26. The classic signs of renal cancer are _____,
_____, and _____.

27. Patients with invasive bladder cancer usually undergo
radical cystectomy and urinary diversion, in which the
ureters are attached to a segment of the _____
to form a _____.

28. The amount of urine left in the bladder after voiding
is called the _____.

29. Manually applying pressure to the suprapubic area to
force urine out is called _____.

30. Three common types of urinary stones are
_____, _____, and _____.

31. _____ stones are the most common
type of renal stones.

32. _____ is a solution commonly used
in stone dissolution.

33. _____ is the surgical removal of a
stone from the renal pelvis.

34. Urethral obstruction secondary to prostatic enlargement is called _____.

35. The only treatment for benign prostatic hypertrophy
is _____.

36. Prostatic massage may be helpful in _____
prostatis, but should be avoided in _____
prostatitis.

37. Medical treatment of prostatodynia is with
_____.

38. In retrograde ejaculation, seminal fluid is discharged into the _____ rather than through the

_____ .

39. _____ is an intrascrotal infection involving the vas and epididymis.

40. A _____ is the most common type of testicular tumor.

41. Pain during urination is called _____ .

42. A lithotrite is an instrument for _____

_____ .

43. Downward bowing of the penis is called _____ .

44. _____ therapy is the first treatment for undescended testis.

45. _____ is a common organic cause of impotence.

46. Surgery to implant a _____ penile prosthesis requires a shorter hospital stay and recuperation period.

47. Secretions from the _____

_____ and _____ increase motility and viability of sperm.

48. Semen analysis evaluates _____ and

_____ of the fluid and _____

and _____ of sperm.

49. Surgery to reverse a vasectomy is called a

_____ .

50. Surgical correction of a varicocele is

_____ .

ANSWERS

1. Cortex, medulla, pelvis.
2. Medulla.
3. Nephron.
4. Glomerulus.
5. Peristalsis.
6. Epididymis.
7. Epididymis, vas deferens, prostatic.
8. Dull, tympanic.
9. Incontinence.
10. Pelvis.
11. Perirenal fat, ureter.
12. Ventral.
13. Pyelonephritis.
14. Renal carbuncle.
15. Enuresis, stress, urge, total.
16. Hematospermia.
17. Hematuria.
18. Diverticulum.
19. Bladder neck contracture.
20. Benign prostatic hypertrophy.
21. Sacral.
22. Detrusor.
23. Cystoscopy.
24. Poor hygiene, intercourse, use of diaphragm.
25. Cystocele.
26. Hematuria, pain, renal mass.
27. Ileum, urostomy.
28. Post void residual.
29. Credé's method.
30. Calcium, uric acid, cystine.
31. Calcium.
32. Renacidin.
33. Pyelolithotomy.
34. Prostatism.
35. Prostatectomy.
36. Chronic, acute.
37. Antispasmodics.
38. Bladder, urethra.
39. Epididymitis.
40. Seminoma.
41. Dysuria.
42. Crushing stones.
43. Chordee.
44. Hormonal.
45. Diabetes.
46. Semirigid rod.
47. Seminal vesicles, prostate.
48. Volume, viscosity, density, motility.
49. Vasovasostomy.
50. Varicocelectomy.

SELECTED READINGS

General references

Dalton J: *Basic Clinical Urology.* Philadelphia: Harper & Row, 1983

Harrison JH, et al, eds: *Campbell's Urology,* 4th ed. Philadelphia: Saunders, 1979

Herman J: *Handbook of Urology.* Philadelphia: Harper & Row, 1983

Kaufman JJ: *Current Urologic Therapy.* Philadelphia: Saunders, 1980

Lapides J: *Fundamentals of Urology.* Philadelphia: Saunders, 1976

Lerner J, Kahn Z: *Mosby's Manual of Urologic Nursing.* St Louis: Mosby, 1982

Luckmann J, Sorensen KC: *Medical-Surgical Nursing: A Psychophysiologic Approach,* 2nd ed. Philadelphia: Saunders, 1980

McConnell EA, Zimmerman ME: *Care of Patients with Urologic Problems.* Philadelphia: Lippincott, 1983

Smith DR: *General Urology,* 10th ed. Los Altos, Calif: Lange, 1981

Winter CC, Morel A: *Nursing Care of Patients with Urologic Diseases,* 4th ed. St Louis: Mosby, 1977

Wyker A, Gillenwater JY: *Method of Urology.* Melbourne, Fla: Krieger, 1975

Chapter 1

Crouch JE, McClintic RJ: *Human Anatomy and Physiology,* 2nd ed. New York: Wiley, 1976

Chapter 3

Assessing Your Patients. Springhouse, Pa: Intermed, 1980

Dalton: *Basic Clinical Urology,* chapter 1

Herman: *Handbook of Urology,* chapter 3

Implementing Urologic Procedures. Springhouse, Pa: Intermed, 1981

Luckmann, Sorensen: *Medical-Surgical Nursing,* chapter 7

McConnell, Zimmerman: *Care of Patients with Urologic Problems,* chapter 2

Winter, Morel: *Nursing Care of Patients with Urologic Diseases,* chapter 2

Wyker, Gillenwater: *Method of Urology,* chapter 2

Chapter 4

Duckett JW Jr: Epispadias. *Urol Clin North Am* 5:107, 1978

Hyndman CW: Congenital anomalies of the genitourinary tract. In Lapides: *Fundamentals of Urology*

Muecke EC: Exstrophy, epispadias, and other anomalies of the bladder. In Harrison: *Campbell's Urology,* Vol. 1

Vaughn E, Middleton GW: Embryology and congenital anomalies. In Wyker, Gillenwater: *Method of Urology*

Chapter 5

Ekelund L, Karp W, Månsson W, et al: Palliative embolization of renal tumors. *Urol Radiol* 3:13, 1981

Lerner, Khan: *Mosby's Manual of Urologic Nursing*, chapter 5

McDougal WS: *Traumatic Injuries of the Genitourinary System.* Baltimore: Williams & Wilkins, 1980

Pollack HM: *Radiological Examination of the Urinary Tract.* New York: Harper & Row, 1972

Pollack HM, Goldberg BB, Morales JO, et al: A systematized approach to the differential diagnosis of renal masses. *Radiology* 113:653, 1974

Wyker, Gillenwater: *Method of Urology*, pages 103-111

Chapter 6

Blaivas JG: The neurophysiology of micturition: A clinical study of 550 patients. *J Urol* 127:958, 1982

Krane RJ, Siroky MB, eds: *Clinical Neuro-Urology.* Boston: Little, Brown, 1979

McGuire EJ, ed: *Urinary Incontinence.* New York: Grune & Stratton, 1981

Stanton SL, Tanagho EA, eds: *Surgery of Female Incontinence.* New York: Springer, 1980

Wein AJ: Pharmacologic approaches to the management of neurogenic bladder dysfunction. *JCE Urology* 18:17, 1979

Chapter 7

Amplatz K: Removing renal stones with fluoroscopic guidance. *Diagn Imaging* March 1983

Chaussy C, Schmiedt E, Jocham D, et al: First clinical experience with extracorporeally induced destruction of kidney stones by shock waves. *J Urol* 127:417, 1982

Herman: *Handbook of Urology*, chapter 17

Kahn R: Nonsurgical technique for removal of upper urinary tract stones. *Contemp Surg* 22:35, 1983

Kaufman: *Current Urologic Therapy*, pages 179-187

Libertino J: *Stones — Clinical Management of Urolithiases.* Baltimore: Williams & Wilkins, 1982

Luckmann, Sorensen: *Medical-Surgical Nursing*, chapter 13

Miller R: New techniques for the treatment and disruption of renal calculi. *Med Eng Tech* 7:1, 1983

Segura J, Patternson D, LeRoy A, et al: Percutaneous removal of kidney stones. *Mayo Clin Proc* 57:615, 1982

Weimerth J, et al: Advances in renal lithiasis. *Urol Clin North Am* 8: 1982

Wyker, Gillenwater: *Method of Urology*, chapter 9

Chapter 8

Burger H, Deretser D: *The Testis.* New York: Raven, 1981

Einhorn LH, ed: *Testicular Tumors.* New York: Masson, 1980

Fraley, EE, et al: Testicular tumors. *Urol Clin North Am* 4:343, 1977

Hafez ES, Spring-Mills E, eds: *Prostatic Carcinoma.* Boston: Kluwer, 1981

Jacobi GH, Hohenfellner RF: *Prostate Cancer.* Baltimore: Williams & Wilkins, 1982

Johnson D, et al: *Testicular Tumors,* 2nd ed. Flushing, NY: Medical Examination, 1976

Peters P, et al: Urologic emergencies. *Urol Clin North Am* 9:2, June 1980

Thompson IM, Carlton C, et al: Genitourinary trauma. *Urol Clin North Am* 4:1, 1977

Chapter 9

Anderson R: Male infertility. In Lapides: *Fundamentals of Urology*

Furlow WL: Male sexual dysfunction. *Urol Clin North Am* 8:1, 1981

Howards SS: Sexual problems in the male. In Wyker, Gillenwater: *Method of Urology*

Malloy TR, Wein AJ: The etiology, diagnosis, and surgical treatment of erectile impotence. *Reprod Med* 20:183, 1978

Von Eschenback AC, Rodriguez DB, eds: *Sexual Rehabilitation of the Urologic Cancer Patient.* Boston: Hall, 1981

Wein AJ, Hanno PM, et al: The evaluation of impotence: University of Pennsylvania approach. In Barrett DM, Wein AJ, eds. *Controversies in Neuro-Urology.* New York: Churchill-Livingstone, 1983

INDEX

Beta-hemolytic streptococcal
infection, 51
Bifid clitoris, 43
Bifid pelvis, 39
Bifid scrotum, 43
Bilateral orchiectomy, 97
Bilateral renal agenesis, 34
Biopsy, 75, 116
Bladder. *See* Urinary bladder
Bleeding tendencies, 21
Bleomycin, 100
Blood flow (renal), 4, 6
Blood pressure regulation, 6
Blood supply
  kidney, 4, 6, 38
  penis, 16, 107, 109
  prostate gland, 13
  renal hypoplasia, 37
  scrotum, 13
  seminal vesicles, 17
  spermatic cord, 16
  testes, 15
  urinary bladder, 10
Blood tests and studies
  impotence and, 109
  kidney lacerations, 54
  prostate disorders, 92
Blunt trauma, 21
  See also Trauma
Bone cancer, 83
Bone scans and studies
  malignant kidney tumor, 49
  prostate cancer, 96
Bowman's capsule, 4, 5
Brain, 69
Brain scan, 49
Buck's fascia, 15
Bulbocavernosus reflex, 109
BUN. *See* Serum BUN levels
Bypass surgery, 109

C

Cadmium, 95
Calcium stones, 82-83
  dietary restrictions, 85-86
  medications, 86
Calculi. *See* Urinary calculi

Calyces (major and minor), 2, 4
Cancer
  impotence and, 108
  kidney, 48-50
  prostate, 95-97
  prostatic massage and, 29
  testicular, 28, 45, 98-100
  urinary bladder, 58, 73-79
  See also Tumors
Carbuncle (renal), 52
Castration. *See* Orchiectomy
Catheterization
  detrusor areflexia, 72-73
  prostatectomy, 93
  prostatitis, 94
  self-catheterization, 62, 65, 70,
    71-73
Cavernous urethra, 11, 12
Cephalexin, 59
Cervix
  assessment of, 29
  exstrophy of the bladder and, 41
Chemotherapy
  malignant kidney tumor, 50
  testicular cancer, 100
  tuberculosis, 53
  urinary bladder cancer, 76, 78
Child birth
  patient history, 22
  stress incontinence and, 63
  See also Pregnancy
Chills
  acute glomerulonephritis, 52
  patient history, 21
  perinephric abscess, 52
  prostatitis, 94
  pyelonephritis, 51
  renal carbuncle, 52
Chordee, 43, 44
Choriocarcinomas, 99, 100
Chronic prostatitis, 94
Cigarette smoking, 74
Circumcision, 44
Cisplatin
  testicular cancer, 100
  urinary bladder cancer, 78
Cleft palate, 41

Hormones
  impotence and, 109
  infertility and, 116, 117
  kidney, 6
Horseshoe kidney, 36, 37
Human chorionic gonadotropin,
    45, 117
Hydration, 51
Hydrocele, 101
Hydronephrosis, 38
  detrusor areflexia and, 72
  ectopic ureter and, 39
  exstrophy of the bladder and,
    41
  hyporeflexia and, 62
  prostatectomy, 93
  prostate disorders and, 92
  ureteral calculi and, 84
  urethral strictures and, 101, 102
Hydroureters, 41
Hydroxyprogesterone, 97
Hypercalciuria, 82-83
Hypernephroma, 48-50
Hyperparathyroidism, 83
Hyperreflexia, 62-63
  medications for, 64
  neurogenic, 70-72
  post-prostatectomy
    incontinence, 66
Hypertension
  patient history, 21
  renal hypoplasia, 37
Hyperuricuria, 83
Hypogastric artery, 15
Hypogastric nerve, 10
Hypoplasia (renal), 37
Hyporeflexia, 62
Hypospadias, 43-44
Hypothalamus, 4

I

Ileoinguinal nerve, 13
Ileostomy, 83
Immunology, 51
Imperforate anus
  exstrophy of the bladder, 41
  urethrorectal fistulas, 45

Imipramine, 64
Impotence, 106-113
  causes of, 107, 108
  erection physiology, 107
  etiology of, 106-107
  evaluation of, 107-110
  nursing implications, 112-113
  patient history, 22
  prostate cancer, 97
  prostatectomy, 93
  treatment of, 110-112
Incontinence
  detrusor-sphincter dyssynergia,
    73
  epispadias and, 43
  exstrophy of the bladder, 41
  hyperreflexia, 63
  patient history, 22
  post-prostatectomy, 66-67
  stress incontinence, 63-65, 67
  urinary bladder disorders, 58
Infantile polycystic kidney, 37
Infection
  Hyporeflexia, 62
  infertility, 117
  kidney, 50-53
  nosocomial, 60
  orchitis, 98
  penis inspection, 28
  prostatitis, 93-94
  testicle, 97-98
  ureteral calculi, 84
  urethral strictures, 101
  urinary bladder, 58-61
  urinary calculi, 84, 85
  urine reflux, 7
Inferior epigastric artery, 13
Inferior vena cava, 6, 39
Inferior vesical arteries,
    7, 10, 13, 17
Infertility, 113-117
  endocrine evaluation, 116
  etiology of, 113
  evaluation of, 113-115
  patient history, 22
  scrotal exploration, 116
  semen analysis, 115-116

Lymphatic system, 99
Lymphoma, 83

M

Major calyces, 2
Malaise
  prostatitis, 94
  pyelonephritis, 51
Male reproductive disorders,
    91-103
  penis disorders, 100-102
  prostate cancer, 95-97
  prostate disorders, 92-94
  testicle disorders, 97-98
  testicular cancer, 98-100
Males
  cystitis, 59
  epispadias in, 42, 43
  exstrophy of the bladder in, 40
  genitourinary tract of, 14
  hypospadias in, 43
  patient history of, 21, 22
  posterior urethral valves, 44
  urethra of, 11-12
  urinary bladder cancer in, 78
Male sexual dysfunction, 105-118
  impotence, 106-113
  infertility, 113-117
Malignancy. *See* Cancer
Meatal stenosis, 45
Meatotomy, 45, 60
Mediastinum testis, 14
Medication
  patient history, 20
  See also Pharmacology; *entries
    under names of drugs*
Medroxyprogesterone, 50
Medulla (renal), 2, 3
Megestrol, 97
Membranous urethra, 11, 12
Metabolism, 108, 109
Metastases
  kidney tumors, 49, 50
  prostate cancer, 95, 96
  testicular cancer, 99, 100
  urinary bladder cancer,
    74, 75, 77

  See also Cancer
Micturition, 9
  See also Voiding
Middle hemorrhoidal artery, 13
Milk-alkali syndrome, 83
Minor calyces, 2
Mitomycin-C, 76
Multicystic kidney, 37-38
Mumps, 98
Myomas (renal), 48

N

Nausea
  acute glomerulonephritis, 52
  patient history, 21
  pyelonephritis, 51
Neonates. *See* Congenital
    disorders
Nephrectomy
  kidney fracture, 54
  malignant tumor, 49
  perinephric abscess, 53
  renal hypoplasia, 37
  tuberculosis, 53
Nephrolithotomy, 88
Nephron, 4, 5
  function of, 4
  structure of, 4
Nephrostomy tube, 86
Nerve supply
  kidney, 6
  penis, 107
  prostate gland, 13
  scrotum, 13
  seminal vesicles, 17
  ureters, 8
  urinary bladder, 10
Nervous system, 108
Neurogenic bladder, 84
Neurogenic disorders, 69-73
Neuromuscular dysfunction, 94
Night sweats, 21
Nitrofurantoin, 59
Nocturia
  bladder neck contracture, 67
  patient history, 22
  prostate disorders, 92

Seminal fructose, 115
Seminal plasma zinc levels, 116
Seminal vesicles, 8, 14, 15, 16-17
    infertility and, 115
    prostatitis and, 94
    spermatic cord and, 16
Seminiferous tubules, 14
Seminomas, 99, 100
Semirigid rod prosthesis, 110-111
Sertoli's cells, 99
Serum acid phosphatase levels, 95
Serum BUN levels
    acute glomerulonephritis, 52
    prostate disorders, 92
Serum creatinine levels, 52
Serum markers, 99
Sex differences
    ectopic ureters, 39
    urinary calculi, 82, 84
Sexual activity
    priapism, 101
    prostate cancer, 95
Sexual dysfunction. *See* Male
        sexual dysfunction
Sexual function history, 23
    See also Patient history
Shellfish allergy, 21
Shock wave lithotripsy, 88
Sickle cell disease, 101
Sitz baths, 94
Skin, 26
Skin lesions, 52
Small-Carrion-type prosthesis,
    110
Sodium bicarbonate, 86
Sperm
    epididymis and, 15
    patient history, 22
    semen analysis, 115
    seminal vesicles and, 16
    testes and, 14
Spermatic artery, 16
Spermatic cord, 13, 14, 15, 16
Spermatic fluid, 12
Spermatogenesis, 113
Spermatozoa, 13
Sphincter urethrae muscle, 12

Spinal cord, 69
Spinal cord injury
    detrusor areflexia, 72
    detrusor-sphincter dyssynergia,
        73
    priapism, 101
Sponge kidney, 83
Stamey procedure, 65
Staphylococcus infection, 52
Steroids
    infertility and, 117
    interstitial cystitis and, 61
    orchitis and, 98
    urinary calculi and, 83
Stone disease. *See* Urinary calculi
Stress
    congenital disorders, 34
    patient history, 22, 23
Stress incontinence, 63-65
    description of, 63
    diagnosis of, 63-64
    post-prostatectomy, 67
    treatment of, 64-65
Struvite stones, 84
Subcapsular hematoma, 54
Sulfisoxazole, 59
Superior vesical artery, 7, 10
Suprapubic bladder neck
        revision, 68
Suprapubic procedures, 65
Suprapubic prostatectomy, 93
Supravesical urinary diversion, 41
Symphysis pubis, 8
Symptomatology
    benign prostatic hypertrophy,
        92
    patient history, 23
    prostate cancer, 95
    prostatitis, 94
    testicular cancer, 99
    urinary bladder cancer, 74
    urinary bladder disorders, 58
    *See also entries under names
        of symptoms*

T

Tabes dorsalis, 72
Tail of epididymis, 14, 15

W

X

OTHER VOLUMES IN THE

NURSING ASSESSMENT SERIES

For information, write to:

Medical Economics Books
680 Kinderkamack Road
Oradell, New Jersey 07649